A voce a mensagem de amor da Casa de
Dom Inácio desejando que os benfeito-
res espirituais o ilumine e ampare

João Teixeira de Faria
PRESIDENTE DA CASA DE DOM INACIO

Spiritual Alliances

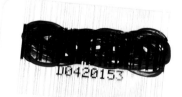

Spiritual Alliances:

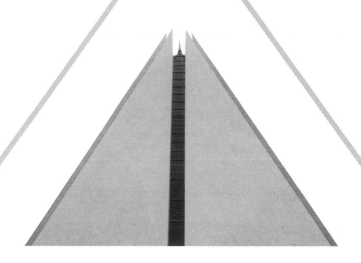

Discovering the Roots of Health at the Casa de Dom Inácio

by

EMMA BRAGDON, PHD.

Lightening Up Press   Woodstock, Vermont

Cover Art: *On the cover is a photograph of a painting completed in 1986 by Luis de Rosário. The painting hangs in the main assembly room at the Casa de Dom Inácio in Abadiania, Brazil. It depicts Christ with his right arm outstretched, his hand overshadowing Dom Inácio de Loyola. In turn, Dom Inácio is guiding the hand of João de Deus who is performing surgery on a patient. The man with the white beard is Bezerra de Menezes, one of the most important founders of Spiritism in Brazil. The man directly to the right of Menezes is Euripedes Barsanulfo. He formerly channeled Menezes as well as Allan Kardec, the author of several books central to Spiritism. The painting depicts both Menezes and Barsanulfo immersed in the flow of energy coming from Christ to Dom Inácio de Loyola and ultimately to João de Deus. Five people in white are meditating to the right of João de Deus, assisting him maintain the energy he needs to do his healing work. The meditators are sitting under a triangle which symbolizes the Trinity: Father, Son and Holy Ghost. The dove over João's head represents the Holy Spirit. A pitcher of water sits on the table. It has been blessed by the beneficent Entities who guide João. Drinking the blessed water is an essential component of each person's therapy at the Casa.*

King Solomon is one of the Entities whom João occasionally incorporates. He is a guiding force of the Casa de Dom Inácio. On the back cover is a drawing of a branch and leaves from a pecan tree, often associated with King Solomon.

Cover Design: *Tom Morgan, Blue Design, Portland, Maine*

Copyright © 2002 by Emma Bragdon, PhD.

Published by:
Lightening Up Press
P.O. Box 325
Woodstock, VT 05091
Phone: 802-457-4915
Email: EBragdon@aol.com

Graphic Design and Layout:
Cookson Desktop Publishing
45 Lyme Road, Suite 204A
Hanover, NH 03755
Phone: 603-643-8858
mark.cookson@valley.net

First Printing: February, 2002
Second Printing: April, 2002
Third Printing: October, 2002
Fourth Printing: February, 2003
Fifth Printing: April, 2004

Manufactured in the United States of America

Main entry under title:
Spiritual Alliances: Discovering the Roots of Health at the Casa de Dom Inácio
1. Health 2. Spiritual Healing 3. João de Deus 4. John of God 5. Casa de Dom Inácio de Loyola 6. Brazil

ISBN #0-9620960-3-2

DEDICATION

This book is a tribute to the extended community which *is* the Casa de Dom Inacio de Loyola. The community is a living example of *spiritual alliances* which improve the quality of life. João Teixeira da Faria contributes his time and energy so that millions may be healed. Staff and volunteers support this work by maintaining the resources of the Casa, and helping visitors from all around the world receive what the Casa has to offer. Highly evolved spirits are available to everyone who comes to the Casa and play an important role in effecting healing. Courageous individuals come to the Casa to request healing and assist others in their healing journeys.

No healer, no spiritual sanctuary, no culture can cure us of our inability to surrender more deeply to love. However, each being we meet, whether he or she is a healer, a person looking for health, or an angel can be an important part of our journey. It is up to each one of us to allow these spiritual alliances into our lives.

Spiritual Alliances: *friendships that empower you to become more integrated, more whole and more aligned with what is sacred.*

ACKNOWLEDGMENTS

This book came to me when I was sitting in meditation and prayer at the Casa de Dom Inácio. I feel that I was gifted with the honor of writing and distributing it. The source of my inspiration needs to be acknowledged—but it is difficult to name that source as it can not be contained in words. The ancient peoples of the Americas have called it— "the Great Mystery." My contemporary friends name it— "the Great Choreographer." Profound thanks to this One.

Angels surround the birth of a child, the birth mother, and the human mid-wives. This book and I have also had a circle of midwives, human and angelic. João de Deus has blessed this book from it's inception—laying his hands on the formal proposal and privately telling me "I will help you with the publication." Six weeks after his commitment the Lloyd Symington Foundation gave me a generous grant to publish the book. God only knows how this is all connected. Celina and Edmund Kellogg, my honorary God-parents, have also helped in inestimable ways through their loving support, including a financial grant. I am honored that you put your faith in me.

Deep gratitude to the courageous souls who come to the Casa for healing—if your stories are not literally contained in this book, they have still been significant contributions to me and I thank you. Special blessings to those who entrusted me to present their stories and their perspectives to the public. It has been a great honor to know you and work with you. May your stories be a contribution to others' healing. I know that is what you want.

I struggle for words to fully acknowledge the people who freely donated their time, their translating skills, their knowledge of Spiritism, and, most of all, their friendship: Joao Ramos, Arthur Santos, and Martin Mosquera at the Casa, and Julika Kiskos and Sylvia Nascimento in San Paulo. Heartfelt thanks to the mediums at the spiritist centers I visited in San Paulo, and the staff and Casa volunteers in Abadiania. You were always there to help me in any way—at your inns, on your faxes and computers, and in every area of the Casa, including the soup kitchen, the juice bar, and the waterfall. The light in your eyes spoke to my heart, even when we didn't share the same language.

The mid-wife who held my hand at the last stage—when I was most weary—was my editor, Joby

Thompson. She lent me her strength, encouraged my soul, and did a great job editing. Joby is one of my Mindfulness Meditation friends who helped me keep my balance while I confronted a maze of decisions.

The circle begins and ends with my family and friends. My parents' capacities as health care professionals and my father's dedication to medical research are perpetual guiding lights. Thank you Marjorie Bragdon, LVN, and Joseph Bragdon, MD. My explorations into unseen worlds *and back* would not be possible without the love and grounding of my son, Jesse Buckley, his wife, Allison, and my extended family.

Illustrations:

Facing page: Judith Ann Griffith
Page 11 – Enzo Bertucci

Photo Credits:

Jerry Howard – pages 22, between 63+64, 89, 102, 112, 137
Mary Kerin – page 59
Karen Leffler – page 3
Jackie Mathey – page 40
Carolyn Morthole – page 136
Rogério – Cover
All other photos by Emma Bragdon

FOREWORD

Brazil declared its independence from Portugal in 1822, and freed its slaves in 1888. Before either of these events occurred, homeopathic medicine was introduced, and a Brazilian spiritual movement evolved in alliance with homeopathy. In 1858, this movement was galvanized by the arrival of *The Spirits' Book* by Allan Kardec (the nom de plume of Leon Hippolyte Denizarth Rivail, a French educator). Kardec's book described a spiritual practice that, for some Brazilians, was more sophisticated and relevant than what they had found in either the African-Brazilian religions or the Roman Catholic church. Kardec's Spiritism (or Kardecismo, as it is called in Portuguese), fostered such doctrines as reincarnation as well as such practices as channeling "spirit guides" in its healing services.

Each of Brazil's many religious traditions boasts stellar healing practitioners. I have observed several of these healers at work, ranging from rain forest shamans to mediums claiming to incorporate "Dr. Fritz," purportedly a deceased German physician. In 1973, I paid my first visit to the Spiritist Federation of Sao Paulo, where my hosts were Jarbas and Carmen Marinho, well known in the Spiritist community for their healing skills and their training programs, including those conducted in Europe. During two dozen subsequent trips to Brazil, I observed many other practitioners, and described their worldviews in several articles and two books.

I am grateful to Dr. Emma Bragdon for this intriguing book about Kardecist Spiritism and the Casa de Dom Inacio de Loyola, named after the Roman Catholic saint who founded the Jesuit Order. Her case studies and interviews provide an important dimension to the ongoing story of Spiritism in Brazil by focusing on the work of Joao de Deus, the dedicated practitioner who has spent several decades attempting to alleviate human suffering.

In 2001, I received a diagnosis of prostate cancer, and opted for external radiation treatment. I also employed several alternative and complementary therapies including Tibetan medicine, homeopathy, "spiritual healing," and the distant ministrations of Joao de Deus. I took herbal capsules he prescribed for me, giving thanks to God and the "healing entities" — those alleged "spirits" who were assisting me. While receiving radiation treatment near my home in California, I also followed Joao's dietary guidelines, which forbade ingesting alcohol, spicy seasonings, and excessive sugar products. The hospital physicians and technicians were pleased that my side effects were fairly minimal; for example, I did not experience the weakness or loss of energy that is frequently reported. After the radiation treatment ended, two follow-up examinations indicated that I was cancer-free. How much did the "healing entities" contribute to the success of this program? I may never know, yet I am extremely grateful for my connection with Joao de Deus.

The associates of Joao de Deus claim to be maintaining records that are already available to serious researchers, including those attempting to unravel the puzzles of "mind/body healing." Dr. Bragdon strongly suggests further investigations of these documents and on-going research on spiritist healing. When this is accomplished, we will look back on Dr. Bragdon's remarkable book and recognize the significant role she played in introducing readers to one of Brazil's unique healers. In the meantime, *Spiritual Alliances* is fascinating to read, and the issues it raises are not only provocative, but profound.

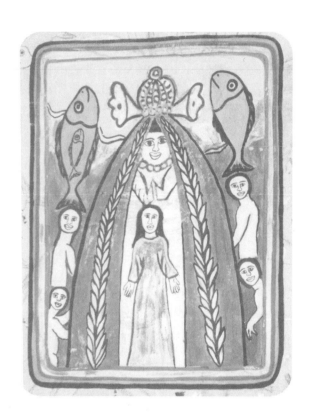

STANLEY KRIPPNER, PH.D.
Alan W. Watts Professor of Psychology
Saybrook Graduate School and Research Center
February, 2002

TABLE OF CONTENTS

PART ONE: BACKGROUND

In November, 1999, Christopher was diagnosed with advanced rectal cancer. He is now cancer-free. The tumor has completely disappeared, without his having had the surgery that the doctors had urged upon him...

In 1995, Sharon, age 35, was diagnosed with arthritis and degeneration of the hip, spine and neck joints —the result of her hip bones being too big for their joint sockets at birth. Among other things, she had tried massage, laser treatment, acupuncture, physiotherapy, Reiki, and herbal supplements. Nothing had turned the tide of the degeneration and increasing pain. Almost all exercise was now impossible. Her regular physicians told her the only thing they could do was do hip replacement surgery. She felt hopeless and depressed. Going to the Casa de Dom Inácio to be cared for by John of God changed her life. She is 80% better now and leads a totally normal life...

Mauro was diagnosed with AIDS in 1993. When he first came to see João that same year his body was covered with sores and he was close to death. In September, 2001 he told me: "I tried one AZT pill, years ago, but it was too expensive for me to continue on it. I never used any conventional medication for AIDS after that one pill. I just saw the Entity, meditated, prayed, and took the prescribed herbs. I never had surgery or used any other treatment at the Casa. For the last seven years I have had no flu, no sickness or any symptoms at all. My physician at home recently said there is no trace of AIDS in my system...

During the two weeks of Dr. Elliott's visit to the Casa de Dom Inácio, she was invited to stand next to the Entity three times, and was asked to report to the audience, as well as live on videotape, what she saw the Entity doing in the visible surgeries. When the Entity scraped eyes with a paring knife, Dr. Elliott, a Board certified family physician, helped him by holding open the eyelids of the patient. Up close, she could see and feel that the patient showed no indication that he was experiencing pain and was not anaesthetized in the conventional sense. She also checked a patient after she watched the Entity cut into the man's abdomen to eliminate a hernia. She reported that there was no evidence of the hernia after surgery...

During the six days he visited the Casa de Dom Inácio in 2001, Frank Salvatore, a Board Certified Urologist, was invited to assist John of God in various healing work. In our interview he said: "We need to increase *the exposure which medical students get to spirit-based healings. Sometimes our indoctrinated beliefs get in the way: We have come to believe that patients can not get well unless they have surgery or drugs; but, sometimes patients can heal themselves without medical intervention from conventional medicine. Where a patient places his or her faith is a potent indicator for healing. Spontaneous remissions do happen. Spiritist healing alone can cure. Prayer can hasten healing...*

The preceding excerpts are typical of the stories gleaned from visitors at the sanctuary in Brazil where João de Deus does his healing work, the Casa de Dom Inácio de Loyola in Abadiania, Brazil. This book tells more about the man, João, and the doctors and patients who visit him— as well as the philosophy behind his work and that of Spiritist Centers. I invite you to consider how our health care system might integrate the successes of such centers.

Outside the Norm: João de Deus

For more than three decades João Teixeira da Faria has had extraordinary success in helping people to heal from AIDS, cancer, paralysis, blindness, mental disease and a host of human infirmities. Some say his success rate is 85%.[1] Although that figure is difficult to concretize, millions of people have consulted with João-in-Entity since 1965. Currently, up to 500 people per day stand and wait in line to see him individually. He continues to have a success rate in his healing work unheard of in western medicine.

This simple Brazilian man, formally educated only through the second grade, is living proof of a unique form of mediumship in which benevolent spirits, aka disembodied entities, or angels, use his body to perform seemingly miraculous healing, including both physical and psychic surgery. When João is acting as a host (to one spirit at a time) he is called "the Entity," and referred to, more formally, as João de Deus (John of God). His intent is to be a vehicle

Dom Inácio de Loyola

for God's work. He has kept to this intention, despite being persecuted and physically abused by those who do not want him to practice his unique way of healing without a medical license.

Brazilians believe that God becomes more accessible through the likes of João and other mediums. They believe that God's energy is too powerful for humans to handle and that, therefore, we need intermediaries, like Jesus Christ, as well as angels, highly evolved spirits, *and mediums* to step down God's energy. Divine energy can thus be adapted to fit our own capacities to receive it, much like an electrical transformer steps down a powerful voltage before it goes into individual homes designed to use weaker voltages.

The Casa de Dom Inácio de Loyola, which houses John of God's work, is one of hundreds of Spiritist centers scattered throughout Brazil. Although John's sanctuary focuses on one gifted medium, most centers are places for charitable work where healing is performed by groups of mediums working together.

In 2001, I visited João's sanctuary for three months because I wanted to see with my own eyes how the Entity could perform successful surgery without causing pain or infection—without anesthesia or antibiotics—relying on help from disembodied entities, spirits or angels. Like many others from around the world, I was drawn by the miraculous and unique nature of João's spiritual alliances. A video I had seen shows him performing surgery blindfolded—to prove that beneficent and highly-skilled forces working through him do the surgery and healing, not João, the ordinary man.

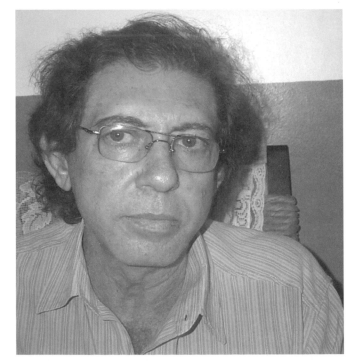

João Teixara de Faria

3

João discovered his gift naturally when he was only sixteen years old. Right from the beginning, he made the commitment to use his what he had been given to serve mankind. His ability to access his gift is amazing—within seconds he can choose to dis-identify with his body and allow a spirit to use it, then re-identify with his body when the work of the spirit is complete. He is an "unconscious medium" because he has no memory of what he does as the Entity.

More than thirty entities, now residing on the spiritual plane, each with his/her own identifiable characteristic personality traits and technical skills derived from former lives as healers, incorporate within João. João-in-Entity diagnoses, offers treatment protocols, confers sedation and operates, prescribes specific alternative therapies, and, sometimes, offers prognoses.

While the Entity consults with individuals who often wait in line for hours to see him, other entities, not incorporated, simultaneously provide healings within the assembled group. In this way, the entities' healing extends to thousands of people a day. Seemingly undaunted by all the attention he gets, João humbly says to the assembled people, "It is not me, but God who does the healing." Neither João nor the Entity ask for any fees for services 'he' renders directly.

Rich and poor, the famous and the forgotten, people of every age come from all over the world to be both inspired and healed by João de Deus at his sanctuary, familiarly called "the Casa," in Abadiania, Brazil. Although many gifted mediums come to support João in his work at the Casa, only João-in-Entity does physical surgery and consults with visitors. Similar to a physician, the Entity accepts responsibility for his patients. Although João de Deus can assume a good deal of authority, e.g. sometimes saying 'I will heal you,' he just as often encourages people to follow their own intuition in making decisions.

Evidence of healing we, in North America, are used to calling "extraordinary," or impossible, is an everyday occurrence at the Casa. During my first visit in the Spring of 2001, I witnessed Anne, a middle-aged French woman with multiple sclerosis, walking by herself after months of being wheelchair bound. I visited daily with David, a man with TB and meningitis whom western doctors had previously predicted would stay a "vegetable," incapable of movement and intellectual acuity. David was socializing more and more each day—talking, participating lucidly in conversation, keeping his head

Dom Inácio de Loyola

4

upright, and deliberately lifting his arms and legs. Elizabeth, my diligent and gracious innkeeper, had been immobilized in bed for eleven years with a brain tumor the size of a grapefruit when she was brought for healing to the Casa. She is now in good health, tending to the cooking, cleaning and laundry for ten to twenty people.

João de Deus has been studied by teams of legitimate scientists from Russia, Germany, the USA, Japan and France.[2] Pathology tests reveal that the tumors, substances and tissues the Entity removes from the sick are indeed human tissues from the individuals operated upon. The most extensive study on João's work lasted two years, was published in Portuguese through a Brazilian university, and made available to the public in 1997.[3] João encourages research into his healing abilities in the hope that medical science can make use of his successes in the treatment of humankind.

Still, it is hard to find a niche for the work that goes on at the Casa. The scientists who studied João are convinced of his capabilities, but bewildered as to how to handle the information. It is very difficult for a scientifically trained mind to comprehend how João is able to perform demanding and complex operations with no medical training. Those trained to believe in the primacy of western medicine like to think of João's work as an unlikely possibility, a "last resort," to be used only after western medicine has "failed."

For those who already believe in the effectiveness of spiritual healing João is not an anomaly, or a last resort, but a dramatic model of what is possible—perhaps *the first place* to turn in a health crisis. The Entity accelerates healing and spiritual growth by nurturing the spirit, where the roots of illness lie.

When we lose our alignment with our spirit and our intuition and we lose our connection to God, we are more vulnerable to disease. Patients under the Entity's care have spiritual experiences which make them more certain of the presence of spiritual realms, the presence of God and benevolent spirits, and the magnificence of their own spirit. They become more motivated to trust in themselves and the world of benevolent spirits, and interested in cultivating spiritual values. Thus, positive participation in their own path to wholeness is encouraged. A positive attitude and a profound spiritual alignment are of inestimable help in confronting illness.

John of God's way of spiritual healing does not attempt to replace western medicine but comple-

"With over 685 deaths per day, this makes conventional medical treatment the third most common cause of death in the U.S."

ments it. When you heal the spirit, you can face sickness and pain with equanimity. When you align your thinking and your behavior with your spirit, you gain peace of mind. Stress diminishes and health is more accessible—even spontaneous remissions of all symptoms can, and do occur.

I believe it is time for more serious research into the effectiveness of both spiritist healing in general and John of God's work, in particular. The findings could affect the lives of millions throughout the world.

The Need for Alternatives in Health Care

In it's "World Health Report 2000," the World Health Organization, WHO, recognized that 36 countries have more successful health care than ours in the USA—even though we are number one in terms of the amount of money spent on health care. Thanks to the scrutiny of world organizations, such as WHO, we can not keep to the limited view that our ways of going about health care will always be the best. Word is out. Doctors, hospitals and consumers of health care are reassessing our way of dealing with health and looking for improvements.

Dr. Dan Fouts recently assessed the effectiveness of our conventional health care: We can pro-

long life through technology. We have excellent emergency medical treatment. We have mapped the genome. However, 120 million Americans have chronic degenerative diseases. Over 50 million more have auto immune diseases. About 90% of medications we use suppress symptoms but do not cure disease.[4] In the early part of the twentieth century medicine made large strides at overcoming infectious diseases through vaccines and antibiotics, but the idea that we are overcoming all illness is a delusion. We can not find vaccines and antibiotics to cure every medical problem.

Our drugs and technology have a shadow side to them. In November, 1998, D.M. Eisenberg and his colleagues published some significant statistics in the Journal of American Medical Association, JAMA.[5] He projected that there are over two million hospitalizations in the USA and more than 100,000 deaths every year, as there have been for the past 30 years, from the expected "side effects" of our pharmaceutical drugs. This, combined with previously documented information that takes into account the mistakes and misuses of pharmaceutical drugs, brings this number to over 5 million hospitalizations, and more than 250,000 deaths annually in the US alone. *With over 685 deaths per day, this*

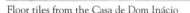

Floor tiles from the Casa de Dom Inácio

makes conventional medical treatment the third most common cause of death in the U.S. This is cause for alarm.

Even the structure of North American health care is inadequate to cope with our needs. The Economist (October 27, 2001) reported that almost a third of the USA's 5,000 hospitals are losing money; 1,000 have closed in the past ten years. Because so many are private, they compete for business. The public health system is in even worse shape. It is understaffed and underfunded. We must expand our health care resources. As a human community we must find a more effective way to manage health care.

The Popularity of the Search for Alternatives

Millions of Americans are finding their own way with complementary health protocols, despite the lack of solid research measuring the safety and effectiveness of alternative and complementary medicine. In response to this grassroots interest in complementary medicine and the proven positive health effects of an active spiritual life, the National Center for Complementary and Alternative Medicine (NCCAM), a division of the National Institu-

tutes of Health, was formed in the 1990s. According to the NCCAM, by conservative estimates, in 1997 over 83 million Americans were consulting complementary and alternative health care practitioners and spending 21.2 billion dollars in the process.[6] It is now estimated that 42% of the U.S. population use complementary medical therapies. *Visits to complementary care practitioners exceed visits to primary care physicians by over 200 million visits per year.* Americans spend an estimated 30 billion a year on these services, the majority of which is not reimbursed.[7] The trend is clear.

What are people looking for? People who go to alternative health practitioners are generally seeking to improve their health and well-being. They want to relieve symptoms associated with chronic or terminal illness or side effects of conventional treatments. Most of these people are not wanting to replace conventional medicine, just complement it with other treatments. Results of a survey about why people gravitate to alternative therapies was published in 1998 in the Journal of the American Medical Association. This study shows that people are finding "an acknowledgment of the importance of treating illness within a larger context of spirituality and life meaning....the use of alternative care is part of a broader value orientation and set of cultural beliefs, one that embraces a holistic, spiritual orientation to life." [8]

Elizabeth Mayer, a psychologist and professor at the University of California's San Francisco Medical School, who also lectures at Harvard and Yale, had profoundly complex problems with her digestive system. Over fifteen years she had consulted with the best physicians in the US as well as highly respected acupuncturists, body workers, medical intuitives, nutritionists, and chiropractors. She went to Abadiania to consult with João de Deus in the summer, 2001. When she left Abadiania she knew there had been a radical change in her. Although she did not receive the "instant cure" she hoped for, she soon came to resolutions which made her problem manageable.

The Link Between Spirituality and Health

Not only are individuals of every stripe now seeking out complementary medical practitioners, but publications of all kinds are covering the subject of complementary health care. The internationally circulated Reader's Digest, never considered a medical journal, ran a special report in September, 2001: "Why Doctors Now Believe Faith Heals—Because they're finding medical evidence". The article pinpoints the positive impact that spiritual experience has on preventing health problems. Among the positive effects of attending religious services was longer life, overall well-being, better recovery after surgery, less likelihood of having heart disease, lower blood pressure, better mental health and reduced levels of stress. Reporter Elena Serocki documented these effects with recent research from leading universities and medical school studies.

Medical students at Georgetown University now have courses that speak to the importance of spirituality for health. (In 1992 only a few of our 125 medical schools had curricula dedicated to religion or spirituality. Now there are 50.) Reghan Foley, a first year medical student, was quoted in saying, "Religion and medicine are inextricably related. We're seeing it time and time again. Everyone has spirituality. It's basically what gives your life meaning." Georgetown Medical School requires students to take "Religious Traditions in Health Care" in their first semester. They cover the correlation between spirituality and health, learning the beliefs of the major world religions from a medical perspective. In this way students are sensitized to culturally diverse issues surrounding euthanasia, transfusion, and the use of technologies to prolong life.

The Need for Research

An important part of the role of National Center for Complementary and Alternative Medicine is to provide the rigorous research needed on various forms of complementary medicine, to advise the public and create standards for research, education and the practice of complementary medicine. NCCAM recognizes that the next step for conventionally trained physicians is to work cooperatively with complementary health practitioners. As of September, 2000, the NCCAM uses the name "Integrative Medicine" to describe this new medical model which combines allopathic medicine with complementary and alternative health care. The work of NCCAM is central to reformulating health care in the US and ultimately creating a replacement for obsolete health-care practices.

I believe that organized, in-depth research of the healing which is promoted through Brazilian Spiritist Centers should be part of our search for improvement. A research project managed over a number of years could verify the elements of success in Spiritist Centers: how they function, what diseases are most often cured, and what part of the population is most effectively served.

Spiritist centers in Brazil are described in the next Part—beginning with my initial experience at the Casa de Dom Inácio and ending with an introduction to Allan Kardec, the man who was the originator of Kardecist Spiritism. Physicians who were invited to be close to João-in-Entity during his work share what they see as the benefits of Spiritist healing for themselves as well as others in Part Three. A few of these doctors were invited and supervised by the Entity to do surgeries at the Casa or assist the Entity in surgical procedures. People who have experienced surgery and healings with João de Deus tell their stories and reflect on the results of the work in Part Four. If you want to know what the culture of the Casa de Dom Inácio is like, and what is expected of you when you are there, read Part Five. In the final section, Part Six, I consider what Spiritist healing and a Brazilian visionary have to offer our more technologically based Western health care. A glossary, notes, resources for additional reading, as well as logistics for traveling to Abadiania from the USA, and finding one's way about the town, are located in the back of the book.

I have interviewed doctors and patients, Casa staff, volunteers and anthropologists. Each perceives the work of the Casa and Spiritism in different ways; each appreciates the gem from a different facet. I leave you to form your own impressions of Spiritism and the work of the Casa, and how they might assist you in your personal health management.

NOTE:

Nothing in this book is meant to replace the advice of a physician. If you have an illness, a mental or physical condition, please recognize the value of seeking many points of view in deciding on a course of treatment. No healer, physician, or disembodied entity who makes him or herself available for our healing, is perfect. Ultimately, the person seeking healing must use his or her best judgment in deciding how to proceed with suggested treatment protocols.

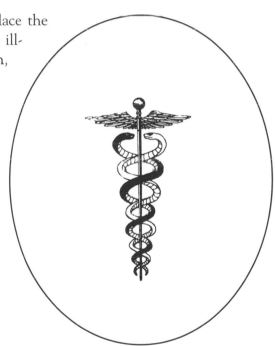

Caduseus

Definition from Webster's Dictionary:
1. *the winged staff carried by Mercury as messenger of the gods*
2. *a representation of this staff used as a symbol of the medical profession*

PART TWO: SPIRITIST CENTERS IN BRAZIL

MY EXPERIENCE AT THE CASA DE DOM INÁCIO

At times, during my initial five week stay in March and April, 2001, I was inches away from João-in-Entity, as he operated with surgical instruments on patients' eyes, noses, stomachs, lower abdomens, and thighs. I saw that he used no visible form of anesthesia or antiseptic, yet people experienced little or no pain and had little, if any, bleeding—clear evidence that something extraordinary was happening. Board certified physicians from the United States witnessed and publicly reported the same to the assembled people and were documented on film. In over thirty-five years of the Entity's surgery, it has been extremely rare for there to be any infections.

My reference points as to what is real and unchanging were altered by what I saw and heard. Somehow, life at the Casa de Dom Inácio operated beyond physical limitations under more powerful spiritual laws. I was deeply fascinated—and sometimes, disoriented as I looked for new reference points.

When the Entity unexpectedly told me I needed surgery, I was surprised. I had no notion that I was physically ill. I chose "invisible surgery," as did most others, including the physicians I interviewed. In the surgery room in mid-March, with thirty-five other people sitting in rows on benches, and a few lying on gurneys, we heard the Entity address all of us, saying a special prayer. He then exited the room, leaving us with his assistants who said additional prayers. A Casa volunteer told me that after the Entity's prayers are said, thousands of healing entities go to work simultaneously attending to the problems of the people in the room.

I put my right hand over my heart during the Entity's prayer. This signaled that I wanted psychological and spiritual healing—to get at the roots of any imbalance I might have. Within seconds, it seemed as if many hands were operating on my heart, removing scar-tissue, renewing and revitalizing the muscle, physically and energetically. I felt a barely perceptible subtle sensation, but no pain. I thought, "Ahhhh, this is removing the effects of separations and deep hurts I have had recently with loved ones." Gratitude and quiet awe filled me on every level. I felt profoundly connected to an invisible spiritual realm where there are many loving beings who enjoy attending the needs of human beings. After 15 minutes or so, the assistants told us the healing session was over.

I did not spend much time doubting my experience—wondering if it was just a product of my imagination, a delusion. I decided to surrender to what I was feeling—and allow the experience to unfold naturally. If, later, I felt the need, I would think about whether or not I had received anything of lasting value.

After the work I felt deep exhaustion, as if I had had physical surgery. It was 10 a.m. and all I wanted to do was sleep, which is highly unusual for me. This need to get extra rest at odd times of the day continued during the length of my initial five week stay in Abadiania. I gave in to it, respecting the notion that some important healing, or psychological integration, was happening while I slept.

During that first visit, in addition to invisible surgery, I experienced the wide variety of healing modalities available at the sanctuary. I had many personal *consultations* with João-in-Entity, some of them dedicated to requesting that he work on people whom I knew who were ill. After my surgery, I was able to act as a surrogate and have the Entity work through me to promote healing for friends and family in Massachusetts, Vermont and California. I spent hours in the "*current rooms*," where one meditates to contribute energy to the entities' work and/or focus on one's own spiritual healing. I visited the *waterfall*, known to assist in purification on a

spiritual level, strengthening good intentions. I had *crystal bed sessions* which balance the energies of the chakras. Every day I drank the *bottled water* which had been blessed by the Entity. I religiously took the *herbal remedies* I had been prescribed. I enjoyed the *blessed soup* given free after morning healing sessions. Above all, I felt the *love* which seems ever-present in the community, where hundreds of volunteers contribute their time and skills to attend to patients.

Before I left Abadiania I was invited to work for the Casa. Catarina Pellegrino-Estrich, an Australian who has worked for the Casa since 1985, encouraged me to become a guide. A number of volunteers asked me to help in facilitating communication between the Casa and the international community. After being inspired to write about the Casa while I sat in current, João-in-Entity gave me his blessing to write this book.

I returned to the casa for another five weeks in August and September—and again for two weeks in December, 2001. I spent as much time as I could in the current rooms, praying and meditating to assist others and clarify my own direction. When I was not doing this work, I took photographs, interviewed people and wrote notes. The initial inspiration I

*"Spiritists deliberately choose to work with spirits who are
highly evolved, exhibiting compassion and wisdom."*

had had, which connected me more deeply to myself and the Casa, deepened into a profound sense of connection and responsibility for our whole world. I committed myself to building bridges of understanding and sharing between Brazil and North America.

Being at the Casa during the razing of New York's Twin Towers and the attack on the Pentagon was simultaneously heart-wrenching and inspiring. I grieved for the loss of life—and the paralyzing fear that now gripped my country. I spent hours in prayer for the political leaders of nations and the executives of major corporations who were taking us toward globalization—"May they allow their hearts and minds to open to deeper levels of service to sustaining the earth's natural resources and supporting the human rights of all peoples." I wanted my prayers to impact all nations intent on making war as a path of conflict resolution. I affirmed a collective vision of all nations appreciating diversity and choosing to live in harmony. I prayed for a spiritual rebirth for all people. Imagine what it would be like if each person primarily experienced him or herself as a soul, transmigrating through births and deaths, evolving toward compassion and wisdom—rather than primarily an individual, identified with a par-

ticular national, religious and racial heritage, seeking retribution and/or competing for material wealth.

During these twelve weeks I noticed changes at the Casa. What initially caught my attention—the dramatic showcase of the Entity's physical surgeries—had given way to more and more Board Certified physicians performing healings in front of the assembled people, under the Entity's supervision. I wondered if the Casa was going to evolve to become an international center—where doctors and healers from many countries learned techniques in healing from the Entity. It seemed as if there were an increasing number of physicians coming to visit.

On my last day in Abadiania, Sonia Maria Teixera Lira, a Brazilian emergency room physician from Rio de Janeiro, and Bob Parker, a North American doctor, worked together while the Entity looked on. I watched Sonia do the eye scraping surgery, where the outer filmy covering of the eye is removed with a paring knife, (thought to be therapeutic for more than twenty one physical conditions in the body) as well as "laying on of hands". She appeared very confident —replacing anesthesia and antibiotics with spiritual anesthesia, prayer, and her own alignment with the Holy Spirit. Her patients at the Casa appeared to place confidence in her, just as they did in the Entity. She was not a novice healer. I can only imagine how she balances her work in a conventional hospital setting with her healing works in a spiritist center. But, she is not unique. There are many physicians in Brazil who are doing just this—the healing work is their volunteer service, contributed for free, on their own time.

Ten months after my initial invisible surgery, I feel a peace of mind which was unknown to me before my trips to Brazil. I still worry about paying my bills, like everyone else, but I hold my worries more lightly, with faith that my life is working and I am doing what my soul was born to do. It feels my life has become much simpler—not complicated by doing what I think others want me to do. It's easier to stick to my deepest sense of purpose and feel that life is supporting me in that. It is also easier to perceive the soul nature of people I know—and not be overly distracted by appearances and reactive judgments. My heart feels open, and, deliciously full of appreciation for life. I know I received spiritual healing at the Casa and I feel deeply honored to be in a position to share the healing work of the Casa with others who may also benefit.

The Casa has its unique path and occupies an important role because the Entity has the intention to contribute to the evolution of health care throughout the world. He demonstrates very clearly that health care must attend to the spiritual roots of disease and dysfunction. The Casa has already welcomed researchers and warehoused thousands of hours of documentary film which are readily available to anyone to view. Most importantly, the Casa provides a contemporary view into the practices as well as the dynamics of a community bonded by sharing Kardec's spiritist philosophy.

Kardec's Spiritism

In the middle of the 19th century Allan Kardec (whose life story is told below) codified the philosophy which became the core of Brazilian Kardecist spiritist centers. Kardec saw some significant differences between Spiritism and Spiritualism — even though they were often confused. In "The Spirits' Book," Kardec wrote:

> "A **Spiritualist** *believes that there is in him something more than matter, but it does not follow that he believes in the existence of spirits, or in their communication with the visible world…*

*A **Spiritist** believes in the existence of spirits, beings of the invisible world, and the notion that they interact in meaningful ways with the visible world. Spiritists deliberately choose to work with spirits who are highly evolved, exhibiting compassion and wisdom."*

A spiritist believes that there is a principle of conscious individuality in each person, a *spirit*, or *soul*, which survives the body. This spirit alternates between a lifetime of learning and a between-lives existence, progressively evolving, until *perfection* is reached. The end goal, the so-called perfection, is a spirit, with or without a body, who is wise, compassionate and happy, and willingly contributes to the transformation of others in their spiritual evolution.

Brazilian psychologist, Julika Kiskos, calls Spiritism "an attitude to life" or "a way of life" for most Brazilians. When a Brazilian is sick, or concerned about a sick family member, he or she often goes first to a spiritist center for assistance. This is a private family affair, as intimately a part of life as eating or sleeping, but rarely spoken about in public, not even to one's religious community or to one's doctor. (Seeing a doctor as well as going to a spiritist center is not seen as a conflict, but a wise way of getting a second opinion.) When a Brazilian comes to live in the United States, he or she sorely misses the spiritist centers. Jacqueline Tyler, a Brazilian licensed as a clinical social worker in North America, told me, "Instead of spiritual life being integrated with physical life as it is in Brazil, spiritual life seems to be held as separate, or even, non-existent in the USA ...When I was twenty and I first got to the USA I thought 'what am I going to do without a spiritist center?' Later, I chose a profession where I could be an active member of Hospice. It seemed to me to be the closest thing you have to the practice of Spiritism in the USA."

Kardec perceived Spiritism as the scientific, philosophical and moral basis of all religions, but not a religion in itself. Kardecist spiritists are benevolent people using principles closely associated to parapsychology, or psychic studies, for healing and spiritual evolution. In addition to attending spiritist centers for consultation and healing work, their spiritual practices include prayer, meditation, charity and the reading of Kardec's books. These practices do not conflict with attending church or having religious beliefs aligned with conventional religions. For the Brazilian people, being a spiritist enlivens spiritual life.

"20% of Brazilians (32 million) regularly attend Kardecist spiritist centers."

> *"What is the true meaning of the word charity as employed by Jesus?"* Benevolence for everyone, indulgence for the imperfections of others, forgiveness of injuries."
> —from Kardec's "The Spirits' Book"

Even though 83% of Brazilians, 133 million, declare themselves Catholic according to the Brazilian Institute of Geography and Statistics, it is estimated that half of these (41.5%) *regularly* attend other forms of spiritual activities. The Federation of Spiritism in Brazil has 2 million registered members and is associated with 6,500 Kardecist spiritist centers in Brazil. "Veja," a Brazilian magazine with a reputation similar to "Time" or "Newsweek," recently wrote that 20% of Brazilians (32 million) regularly attend Kardecist spiritist centers.[1]

It is likely that 80% of Brazilians use the resources of spiritist centers for assistance *at some point in life* when they are in need of healing, participating in some form of spiritual group gathering which involves mediums. Slaves who survived the trip from Africa, numbering 10 million from 1459 to 1853, imported a tradition of working with spirits in religious ritual. As a result of intermarriages Brazilian culture was infused with mediumistic religions and philosophies. Brazilians who are spiritists can choose from *Candomble*, derived from African roots, *Umbanda*, originating with native Brazilian Indians, or Kardecist Spiritism.

Part of being a Brazilian Catholic typically involves many forms of religious and spiritual expression. Attending Mass may happen on Sundays, or high holidays, or not at all. Brazilians love to pay homage to an indigenous female aspect of God, Iemanja, by throwing flowers and fruits into the sea at specific times and places, close to the New Year. This is one way to please the mother of the waters, gain protection and good luck. Figurines which incorporate the spirits connected to Umbanda are kept in many households to proffer good fortune. Attending a spiritist house for healing, or to consult with a medium who can facilitate communication with a dead relative, are also not unusual activities for Brazilian Catholics.

Despite the apparent philosophical flexibility of most Brazilian lay people, Catholic and Christian church *authorities* rarely endorse Spiritism. These are the reasons: spiritists believe in reincarnation and the evolution of each spirit over lifetimes, which almost all forms of Christianity dismiss. Spiritists allow people to participate in channeling and or receiving the Holy Spirit, even exorcising a negative spirit, without the intervention of a priest authorized by the church. (Authorities of the Catholic church and evangelical Christians, even some fundamentalist Kardecist spiritists, liken psychic surgery to the work of a witch doctor, "curandeiro," and try to obstruct people like João from performing surgeries.)

Spiritists believe that miraculous healing can be attributed to natural psychic phenomena; that angels and demons are only more or less highly evolved spirits; that heaven and hell are within us. Our response-patterns to life create heaven or hell —we make ourselves happy or unhappy. Thus, heaven and hell are psychological constructs, not physical places as the Bible suggests.

How was it that Brazilians allowed Kardecist Spiritism, a philosophy born in France in the middle of the 19th century, to come so close to their religious philosophy in the first place? Brazil was fertile ground for Kardec's brand of Spiritism because it already had a rich tradition of spirit-mediumship religion, where mediums are used to link with spirits who are not in body as part of religious ritual. These religious rituals originated with the African slaves and the Native South American Indians, and had never been completely suppressed by the church. These ancient practices might include "black magic,"

or using spiritual powers to hurt others. They are referred to in a pejorative way by the Kardecist's, who call them "Quimbanda," or "Macumba," similar to the English generic term,"voo-doo".

Brazil's receptivity to Spiritism can also be traced back to homeopathic physicians who were in Brazil using homeopathic remedies and "magnetic healing" (a form of energy healing) just a decade before Kardec's writing gained notoriety.[2] These homeopathic doctors were already working with the poor for free, often diagnosing and choosing homeopathic remedies using intuition seasoned with their scientific training. The emphasis on energetic healing, charity, prayer, listening for spiritual guidance through intuition and their own sense of spiritual evolution fit hand in glove with Kardecist Spiritism. In 1848, nine years before Kardec wrote the "Book of Spirits," the first Brazilian spiritist group was founded. When Kardec's book arrived in Brazil in 1858, it generated even more interest and strengthened the already existing spiritist groups linked to homeopathy.

In sum, it appears that the Brazilians who took to Kardec's Spiritism let go of any semblance of negative intent in the spiritual mediumship traditions of their country while holding fast to the notions of reincarnation and the positive potential in spirit communication. Kardec's doctrine added the concept of spiritual evolution and the law of cause and effect (similar to karma),to these basic elements, and deleted all ritual. Thus was born a way of life which asked people to act with charity towards each other, stay open to a helping hand from beneficent spirits, and directly receive or learn to channel the healing energy of God.

Kardecist Spiritist Centers in Brazil

Profoundly moved by what I had seen in Abadiania, I wanted to understand more about Kardecist Spiritism. In August, 2001, I visited three spiritist centers in San Paulo which are more typical of most other spiritist centers in Brazil. This allowed me to see the Casa de Dom Inácio from another point of view, in context with other spiritist centers.

The Kardecist spiritist centers I visited in San Paulo do not have a charismatic leader, like João, who performs surgery and prescribes herbs. Instead, the healing work is done through energetic "passes," where the energy of the Holy Spirit is channeled by trained mediums working in teams of two to five people. Similar to "laying on of hands," the body of the patient is not touched. The healers do not give consultations, diagnoses or prognoses. These same mediums may, at various events during the week, offer automatic writing, perform healing at a distance, or channeling of elevating words to inspire a greater understanding of spiritual evolution, but the healing sessions are simply dedicated to transmitting the energy of the Holy Spirit.

In general, all spiritist centers have an important role in building and maintaining community. They often function as an extended family, providing love and safety as well as healing. This is especially important now when Brazil's cities are known world-wide for their poverty and lack of safety. Seven thousand people a day come to the Federation of Spiritism in San Paulo and use the services of healing, child care, kindergarten, free soup, a library, lectures, artistic and musical productions, parenting classes, sewing and knitting, and consultations with doctors, homeopaths, dentists or financial planners. These are provided free to families in need of such social services. Two thousand mediums work at this center on a voluntary basis. The centers survive by donations. They are not sponsored by the government or any religious organization.

Many spiritist centers offer classes on Kardecist Spiritism for adults and, separately, for teens as well. *Spiritism is presented as a way of life, not a religion.* Students learn the nature of cause and effect, the importance of thinking positively, the nature of spiritual evolution, and how to lead a moral life. Performing acts of charity and being unselfish are central to spiritist values and, in this way, Spiritism is essentially harmonious with Christianity (and many other religions).

Volunteering at a center allows people to practice charity in a variety of ways. It might include donating money, making and serving soup, teaching classes, doing healing or office work, or any of the various maintenance jobs which are necessary in maintaining a center. Through charity they make amends for things they did in the past which were not motivated through compassion. Through charity they accelerate their spiritual evolution.

CHÁ ARTESANAL

Selling herbs

If spiritist centers are so well frequented in a country of 160 million, why haven't we heard more about it? Brazil was under military rule or dictatorship from 1930 until 1989. In the 30's and 40's the government tried to repress all activities associated with Spiritism. In the 1990's, increased freedom of the press came hand in hand with unpredictable economic problems. There has been little money dedicated to formally quantify the success of spiritist healing. An individual, like João, practicing surgery with no medical license, represents a political nightmare. The Catholic church, the medical profession and the government all have a vested interest in overlooking the positive impact of his healing work—it challenges the authority of science, religion and government licensing laws. Similarly, other spiritist houses are perceived as threatening the authority of medical science and conventional religion.

In light of these complex political, economic and social issues, spiritist centers devote their resources to helping people in the here and now. They keep a low profile and do not proselytize. They do not have extra storage space to quantify data, secretarial staff to manage extensive records, or expensive computer services and research teams. The only downside of this focus is that the successes of

"Man acts rightly when he takes the good of all as his aim and rule of action…"

spiritist healing centers remain largely invisible. Statistics which enumerate the number of people involved and their success stories are difficult to find.

Medium's Training

One of the most amazing resources of spiritist centers in Brazil, little known in North America, is "Medium's Training." This is training in managing and developing one's psychic abilities (modes of acquiring knowledge without being cued by external senses) for the purpose of healing work. It may or may not include incorporating entities. The training takes at least four years to complete. It includes cognitive understanding as well as practical skill building. This special training is offered in some, not all of the spiritist centers.

The Brazilian Spiritist Federation (FEB) has published the books which are used in the training of mediums. These include books by Kardec, which have also become available in English and on the web (See resources at the back of this book). Some of the books most often used in this training, like "Missionarios Da Luz" (Missionaries of Light) by André Luiz, have not yet been translated into English.

After training, graduates, now formally referred to as "mediums," work together in teams. As mentioned earlier, this teamwork provides a way to practice charity by being an agent of healing for others. Sharing the work also helps the medium's avoid becoming egotistical because they share the responsibilities and the successes of the healings. At least once a year, the mediums are monitored by a senior practitioner and given feedback on their ability to stay balanced and strong in their work. If they refuse to lead a moral life, or they can not put their selfish desires aside in order to work clearly in service of others, the mediums are asked to stop working as healers. All told, medium's training contributes to mental health as it strengthens mental focus, creates teamwork, instills habits of being in service to others, and supports each person in being deliberate with his or her natural psychic abilities.

Spiritists believe that everyone is a "medium." We might translate this as: every human being is born with some psychic abilities, or special sensitivities, aka extra-sensory perception. There is no word for "psychic" in Portuguese. Brazilians find it strange to consider a person with psychic abilities as out-of-the-ordinary.

Spiritists also believe in the value of harnessing psychic abilities. If we don't use them deliberately, in a positive manner, they can work against us and be a component of psychological disorders. Kardec, in fact, wrote that 70-80% of mental illness originates in people not knowing how to manage their psychic abilities. The idea that each person has within him/her the potential for spiritual healing, psychokinesis, precognition, or one or more other psychic abilities is quite new to our North American culture. Although Larry Dossey, MD., in "Healing Words," writes that more than three decades of high quality research has been conducted which confirms the existence of psychokinesis (mind over matter), and precognition; in North America, we are only just beginning to explore how to teach people to recognize and harness these potentials.

Could it be true that not using these psychic abilities contributes to mental illness? Imagine a plant trying to break ground and grow toward the sunlight. If a rock is placed over the spot it is breaking ground—the growth will turn back into itself. The shoots that could have been tall and straight, producing green leaves, flowers, or vegetables, become white, leafless, ingrown and matted. Perhaps the same is true of people gifted as mediums in our society. If we deny the reality of the spirit world and rarely give a respectable position to those who claim to communicate with spirits, we may stunt or obstruct the growth of mediums. In this case, it would be natural for many of our people gifted with psychic abilities to respond by turning back on themselves and growing in on themselves with obsessions, compulsions, unnecessary anxieties and depression.

Seen from this vantage point, the mediumship training offered in spiritist centers serves two important purposes which have immense significance in society: 1 skill building to assist in healing others and 2. *maintaining mental health*. Teachers of these classes have years of interaction with their students, providing on-going structured support as well as assisting students in finding an outlet for their abilities which benefits the community. Said in another way, people who formerly may have had mental "problems" are put on a track where they are more and more identified with personal growth, enhancing their capacity to serve the greater good. Lack of willpower, a weak sense of direction, and the self-centeredness which often accompanies mental illness is transformed into mental health and charitable works. What would be considered a "treatment protocol" in one lexicon becomes a path of continual growth in another. The result is less mental illness, more people functioning as healers, and more networks of support. (Quite an alternative to med-

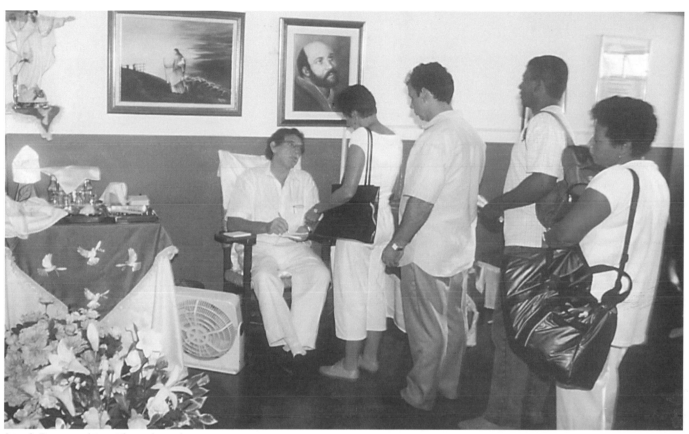

João de Deus consulting with people one by one

ical diagnoses which undermine self-esteem and encourage a negative self-image; and psychiatric medications which are expensive and often have negative side-effects on the nervous system and liver.)

If some illnesses are indeed karmic (meaning a person is paying for past transgressions towards others through the currency of suffering mentally or physically) then this treatment is a direct path from the suffering due to bad karma, to good karma.

> "*In order to insure our future happiness, is it sufficient not to have done evil?* No; it is necessary for each to have done good also, to the utmost limits of his ability; for each of you will have to answer, not only for all the evil he has done, but also for all the good which he has failed to do....Man acts rightly when he takes the good of all as his aim and rule of action..."
> —from Kardec's, "The Spirits' Book"

Let's look at an illustration of how this point of view might help us manage mental health problems in health care professionals. Consider the fact that doctors and mental health professionals are often drawn to their professional work because they have compassion and want to help others. In their professional life, consulting with numbers of people who are suffering, they become increasingly more able to sense the energy of particular moods in their patients, for example, depression—and increasingly saturated with negative energy from patients who are suffering from negative states of mind and/or body. Over time, like a sponge, they absorb these energies. Yes, this may enhance empathy, which is good. However, this *clairsentient psychic ability* (the ability to feel others pain without verbal or physical cues), if left unmanaged and unconscious, may be a leading cause of suicidal depression, alcoholism and drug abuse in doctors and psychologists. Imagine a sponge that is fully saturated. Clairsentience can make health care workers so absorbed in the energy of their patients, they lose their ability to clearly differentiate their own feelings and perceptions from those of others. This may be one reason physicians have the shortest life expectancy of any profession. Medium's training can help health professionals be empathic, and, at the same time, able to deliberately let go of negative energy and fill themselves continuously with positive energy.

Now that we have understood and appreciated the flowering of Kardec's Spiritism, let's go back to the man himself, to see how this French educator came to create the philosophy for a social movement which has been, and remains, so important to the people of Brazil.

Allan Kardec

The way in which Kardec's books came to be written is, in itself, a mark of the extraordinary. The name, Allan Kardec, was assigned as a "nom de plume" by the spirits who oversaw the writing of the book. The real man, Leon Denizarth Rivail, was born to a family of lawyers in 1804. From a young age Rivail had a passion for teaching. By the time he was 24 he was head of a boy's school, giving well-attended public lectures on themes related to theoretical mathematics, linguistics and the improvement of public education. He was also involved with the Phrenological Society of Paris and active with the Society of Magnetism where he researched clairvoyance, among other things. Around 1850, he was introduced to two mediums who, in Rivail's company, began to channel spirits of a high order who were there to "enable him to fulfill an important religious mission."

Rivail, not a medium himself, relied on the talents of the two mediums for his communication with the spirits. Rivail asked questions and recorded the answers. The resulting *Spirits' Book* was then published and became highly popular in western Europe. Over the next few years Rivail and others formed associations all over the world for the purpose of obtaining from spirits further clarification about truth and the purpose of life. Rivail, in his role as president of "The Parisian Society of Psychologic Studies," received the most remarkable of these spirit-communications, sent to him from other groups who wanted to contribute to the work. He collated and organized these communications—revising *The Spirits' Book* (1857), and compiling four other works: *The Mediums' Book* (1861), *The Gospel as Explained by Spirits* (1864), *Heaven and Hell* (1865), and *Genesis*, (1867). Rivail died in 1869.

Surprisingly, Kardec's books are well-known in Brazil, but he remains a virtual unknown in North America. Brazilians I met were shocked that I didn't initially know Kardec's name and hadn't read his books. (How could I have a doctorate in transpersonal psychology and not know Kardec,? they wondered.) My ignorance was a reflection of our North American prejudice against Spiritism. We have regarded it as a cult activity associated with voodoo, rather than a useful complement to religious life.

Recent generations of Brazilians continue to gravitate to Kardec's Spiritism. They find it lends vitality to spiritual life and is easy to practice alongside conventional religion.

Are North Americans ready to consider the possibility that Spiritism may provide something of value to our religious and spiritual life, as well? Certainly, spiritist doctrine can clarify some issues which religions have obscured, and spiritist practices can revitalize our connection to our spiritual roots. Kardec felt that Spiritism would revitalize Christianity!

PART THREE: SPIRITS AND DOCTORS

As a child I was aware of the fence separating Spiritism and Science. I got a view into the field of conventional medicine through my father, a brilliant research pathologist who worked at the National Institutes of Health. I got a peek into a generic form of Spiritism through two of my aunts each of whom had a compelling interest in psychic phenomena. The barrier separating these two fields seemed impenetrable. In my family it was taboo to speak of them both in the same conversation. Mealtime conversation was limited to a certain standard of intelligence, measured by my father's loyalty to science.

There was no opening which would allow a flow of movement or an exchange between the two fields. Psychic phenomena, like spirits, were relegated to ghost stories for scaring friends at night, parlor games to occupy children who had nothing better to do but be frivolous, or very private conversations which would remain secret. Those who spoke of spirits in public opened the door to being perceived as foolish or crazy. In such a world, doctors were more than real, rightfully deserved authority and assumed great responsibility. Speaking of medicine and helping people who were suffering from physical problems was serious and allowed no room for any-

thing which might be perceived as unscientific. This separation of science and psychic phenomena is still quite common in the United States.

I was twenty years old, and already intent on studying the psychology of higher states of consciousness, before I heard of Edgar Cayce and J. B. Rhine. Cayce (1877-1945) was the first anglo-North American who had impressed physicians with his diagnostic skills...skills which were accessible to him through communicating with a spiritual intelligence. Cayce could deliberately put himself in a "sleep state" to channel spirits. Although he was not educated as a doctor, in his sleep state he successfully diagnosed and gave treatment plans for the ill or emotionally disturbed, as well as inspired people to deepen their spiritual lives. His successes are well documented and his work is still studied at the Association for Research and Enlightenment in Virginia Beach, VA, founded in 1931.[1] However, Edgar Cayce was never recognized as more than an anomaly. Our collective belief systems have no place to put a person like a Cayce or a João de Deus, who straddle the fence between medicine and Spiritism.

J.B. Rhine was the first North American to bring parapsychology into the laboratory for research. His work began in the 1930's at Duke University where he did double blind studies on mental telepathy and other psi phenomena, raising psychic studies to a science. Since then thousands of studies have been done on subjects related to parapsychology. Many have been completed in labs which employ our best thinkers, such as Stanford Research International and Princeton which hold to the highest standards of research. Still governmental bodies, like the National Research Council, which shape public opinion, prefer to overlook many of the outcomes of this excellent research and thus, through inaction, support our culture's habit of not recognizing the contributions of parapsychology in health.[2]

Perhaps my introduction to the world of spirits was like yours. In 1954, our family was given a Ouija board. I was eight years old at the time; my sister and her friends were fourteen and fifteen. We would take the board out in front of the fireplace on chilly winter nights. The Ouija board was, after all, considered a "parlor game," and was sold next to other board games like "Monopoly" and "Parcheesi".

The Ouija board itself is a piece of particle board with the alphabet and numbers 1 to 10 printed on a smooth paper on one surface. It comes with a plastic device an inch high and five inches wide standing on three felt-tipped legs so it can easily glide on the surface of the board. This gadget has a window in it's center so you can view an area of the board through it. We would gently rest our hands on the device after it was placed on the center of the board. With no intent, or prayer, or ceremony, we would wait for it to be moved by spirits. When the three legged viewer became animated, as it usually did, it would slide around the board, stopping over a letter of the alphabet or a number. My hands remember this feeling of surrendering.

We did our best to follow the instructions given in the game box: let go of control and allow the device to be moved by a different energy than your own. We hoped *some* spirit would be there. When it moved we either prodded each other, "Are *you* pushing it? Are you...?" or kept an awed silence. We recorded what we saw on paper and then pieced together the message that was "coming through" from the spirit realm. Most of the questions centered around "Does so-and-so like me?," or "How many children will I have when I grow up?" (We could have just as easily asked a daisy...He loves me, he loves me not, he loves me, he loves me not.)

We played this game mindlessly, waiting for dinner to be ready. When we received coherent messages, we laughed. The names we received were so strange, the messages somehow unbelievable. I don't remember any discussions about the real origin of these energies we were contacting, or of how we could use the board as a medium to really benefit someone. No one knew to warn us that if spirits came through to us, they could have had a less than benevolent intent. Ignorant, we opened the door to *all* spirits—just as a child might leave the front door of a house open for anyone to walk in. We didn't know how to be selective. We didn't know we *should* be selective. We played the game—just to have fun.

My introduction to the notion of communicating with spirits continued in this haphazard way, interspersed with ghost stories and odd dreams of American Indians coming to take me away from my parents' home. Psychic phenomena were part of my life through my own gift of clairsentience. I seemed to have a keen sense of recognition about what was really going on with others. Even though my parents pretended to be cheerful around me, I knew that each of them was suffering profoundly—I palpably felt the depression.

When I was alone with my Aunt Celina, driving in a car or having a cup of tea, she shared stories with me about her experiences with "the other side." In the early 1940's she and a few other women had gathered around a table in Boston for seances, hoping the greater intelligence of those in the spirit world might tell them about their husbands who were away in the war in Europe and Asia. Mail came rarely and information was never enough as the men were not allowed to tell their wives where they were and what they were doing. During the seance each woman laid her hands on the table with the intent of communing with spirits —asking specific questions about family and friends. The table legs, without being lifted physically, responded to the energy of disembodied spirits, and thus tapped out letters of the alphabet arrived at by the number of taps. A=1 tap, B=2 taps, C=3 taps, etc. One evening Aunt Celina's dead grandfather identified himself, saying he approved of the fact that his grandson, Henry, was choosing to join the ministry, and assuring everyone that Henry was all right. Aunt Celina told me that this seemed so real and honest, she stayed awake, dazed, most of that night. Gratefully, Henry did survive the war and went on to become a well-loved Episcopal minister. Another night the table became so animated, the women were chasing it as it walked upstairs by itself. The table was insistently tapping the letters A-H-F, A-H-F, A-H-F. They didn't understand the meaning of the message until the phone rang the next morning with word that a cousin, Augustus Horsford Fiske (A.H.F.), had died unexpectedly.

These stories were told to me with a "we better not take this too seriously" attitude (most of the men in our family were physicians who had been trained in the best medical schools in the country) but the stories hooked me on a much deeper level. I wanted to know more about these phenomena.

I also felt especially connected with my mother's sister, Aunt Harriet, or "H," who also had a determined interest in spiritual questions. From 1955-1967, H. met once a week with a small circle of women (including a woman who communicated with evolved spirits) to study the great books of perennial wisdom: the I Ching, Tibetan Book of the Dead, the writings of Jung, the Bible, etc. They started their meetings by meditating together in silence. At the end of these meetings, the woman who channeled the spirits sometimes offered wisdom from her disembodied sources.

H's group grew socially active and contributed to the growth of new spiritual practices in the US. It was not simply a support group for a small number of women. In 1965, members of this group brought Philip Kapleau back to the USA to be a meditation teacher in Rochester, NY, after his years studying in Japanese monasteries. Kapleau later wrote "The Three Pillars of Zen," a classic in the literature of Buddhism in America, and became a highly revered teacher in the US. Thus, I hold my Aunt H as a real leader in support of Americans opening to new and powerful forms of spiritual work aimed at implementing enlightened ways of life.

Where my aunts were a source of inspiration, inviting me through an opening into the vast field of spiritual inquiry, H's husband, Bill, and my father did everything to close that opening. I noticed that my mother and her sisters were predictably silent about psychic phenomena and the wisdom traditions in the company of their men. At first I didn't understand why. So, as a teenager, I asked Bill and my father for points of view on the invisible realm of spirits and meditation teachers. Bill thought meditation was for the birds, parapsychology was unreal, and metaphysics was not for people who had any brains at all. Bill teased H. mercilessly and publicly about her study group. He saw no value in what he called "staring at your navel," or "cloud meetings."

My father (who trained at Johns Hopkins Medical School in the 1930's, and taught at Harvard Medical School before his employment as head of a research laboratory at the National Institutes of Health) summarily dismissed any health professional who gave weight to the power of an invisible energy—"Must be a quack," he would say, or "a snake oil salesman." When I had the courage to ask my Dad about chiropractic or acupuncture or meditation he would reject the subject and me in less than two seconds. It was a quick lesson.

Bill's and my father's reactivity and closed-mindedness impressed upon me the need to be very cautious about who you speak to about psychic phenomena. Talk about anything related to the invisible world and you just might lose your friends, even your family's love and your credibility in a flash.

Despite the well-documented medical successes of Edgar Cayce, as well as others like him, spiritist healing is still maligned in the Western world as being no more than parlor games, hocus-pocus, hypnosis or the placebo effect. The Journal of American Medical Association will have nothing to do with Spiritism, as if the successes of this kind of healing don't exist. Although we will probably not be burned at the stake in the 21st century North America, those who believe that spiritual practices can effect healing can still be skewered by the intelligentsia and discounted by medical authorities.

We have become the hostages of a vast act of profanity, predominant in the scientific and technical paradigm. This sacrilege has reduced the universe to a mechanical and mathematical inert reality and the Earth regarded as a simple repository of resources made available to the human race.

—Leonardo Boff, Brazilian theologian, December, 1998, "*Brazil*"

It is sad to see the effects of the unyielding prejudice of our medical system toward anything related to Spiritism. We deny a variety of effective healing procedures and human potentials. We also insult the intelligence of other cultures who have been successful using spiritist healing as part of health management.

Why is it that anatomists, physiologists and in general, those who apply themselves to the pursuit of the natural sciences, are so apt to fall into materialism? "The physiologist refers everything to the standard of his senses. Human pride imagines that it knows everything, and refuses to admit that there can be anything which transcends the human understanding. Science itself inspires some minds with presumption; they think that nature can have nothing hidden from them."

—from Kardec's "The Spirits' Book"

Fortunately, a rebirth of interest in altered states of consciousness is well under way, and with it a new look at all things spiritual. Channeled books authored by spirits have gained considerable notoriety in the last few decades. *A Course in Miracles*, penned by Helen Shucman who claimed to be channeling Jesus, has fostered study groups in 14 languages, and sold approximately one million copies since it was written in 1965.

More recently doctors like Larry Dossey have published research showing the healing power of what has previously been dismissed as unreal. We now know that a strong spiritual life contributes to mental health and longevity. People who believe in God or a Higher Power, attend church, and regularly pray have more satisfaction in life and more emotional stability. Dr. Dossey has collected evidence on the efficacy of distant prayer in healing.[3] The Journal of Alternative Therapies, of which Dossey is Editor-in-Chief, published an article in July, 2000 on "Trance Surgery in Brazil," by N. Don and G. Moura, the first to suggest, albeit superficially, the positive power of psychic surgeons in Brazil.

Thus, some brave souls are walking between the fields of medicine and Spiritism, trying to illuminate how we can engage both together, at least have them converse. Ease of travel is assisting these efforts. We live in a time where individuals have the freedom to visit the Casa de Dom Inácio to experience spiritist healing, as well as have access to life-saving technology and drugs originating in our finest research laboratories and hospitals.

> *"Why has not the Truth been always placed within reach of everyone?* Each thing can only come in its time. Truth is like light; you must be accustomed to it gradually; otherwise it only dazzles you."
>
> – from Kardec's "The Spirits' Book"

Fortunately, I was able to make a contribution toward North Americans accepting the possibility that psi phenomena are not indicative of mental illness. In 1986 I completed my Phd in Transpersonal Psychology. A portion of my dissertation, "A Sourcebook for Helping People in Spiritual Emergency," was later published as a book and is now used in some graduate school programs. This work, along with that of many others, became a factor contributing to psychiatrists re-evaluating the symptoms associated with psychosis. By 1994 the Diagnostic and Statistical Manual of Mental Disorders included a new diagnostic code, "Religious or Spiritual Problem" to label those issues related to the disorientation which comes with spiritual growth that do not indicate mental illness. Since this inclusion, therapists and health professionals are responsible for discerning the difference between extraordinary spiritual experiences and symptoms of mental disease. It is a step towards breaking away from our cultural prejudice and ignorance regarding psi phenomena, and spiritual experiences which can initiate significant healing.

As discussed in Part Two, Brazilians are ahead of us in accepting the power of spiritual healing. Spiritism has deep roots in the culture, and continues to grow in contemporary society. Chico Xavier, a well-known Kardecist spiritist from Uberaba, now in his 90s, transmits the wisdom of highly evolved spirits to thousands of people everyday. His hand is animated by a spirit who can diagnose and suggest treatment for people seeking healing. He has channeled over three hundred books, in Portuguese, all testifying to the power of the healing possible when we interact with spirits in the correct manner. Brazilians consider him a living saint. He has been nominated for the Nobel Peace Prize.

Still, as western science and technology makes its way into Brazil, the wisdom of Spiritism is being challenged. A Brazilian licensed psychologist who practices healing at a distance through prayer, or depossession of negative spirits for the benefit of her clients, can lose her license in Brazil just as quickly as a psychologist in the USA who uses the same protocols in her practice.

Do we weaken our practice of medicine by isolating ourselves behind our rational, scientific paradigm? What happens to those who remain solidly fixed in the old paradigm of Western science? Unfortunately my father died of heart failure, alone and disconnected from family. He was only 58 years old when his heart stopped in 1972. I think he had put more stock in his well-trained mind than in his heartfelt connections. Ironically, my father's specialty back in the 50's and 60's was heart disease. He championed the materialist's point of view: don't clog the arteries with too much fat and your heart pump will keep doing its job. A valuable perspective at the time—but not the whole story.

Currently, thirty years after my Dad's death, medicine recognizes that support groups where people share their stories and retain close connections with each other are at least as important for the health of the heart—as diet and exercise. Heartfull connections, that invisible stuff which allows us to commune with each other and become allies in spirit, is finally being recognized in the practice of medicine.

What happens to our medical institutions when we remain solidly fixed in the old model of Western science and don't restructure them to adapt to the importance of human connectedness? Our hospitals purchase more and more technology. Our researchers try to duplicate the stuff of life, mapping the genome, cloning animals, *without answering the question of what gives life meaning*. Doctors and psychologists have less and less time to develop supportive, authentic relationships with patients and, thus, relate only through the techniques they offer: surgery, anesthesia, cardiology, etc. As technologists, intent on holding on to life, we become islands unto ourselves, separated from a vast sea of connections, even separated from being "at one" with ourselves.

Even though we are considerably more open to alternative or complementary medicine now than we were in the 1950s; we still have to deal with our attachment to the indoctrination we have received, and the way our medical institutions are structured. For example, we hold on to life using extraordinary means to maintain it even when there is no longer any hope of a life of quality. Today, a dying person is still typically surrounded by the technology of medicine to the point where large machines for life support and the nurses who monitor them become the central point of focus. Immobilized by tubes and overstimulated by noise—the critically ill person does not have the peace of mind to meditate or make peace with his God, even if he wants to. The Hospice movement has helped us get around this paralyzing situation by taking our loved ones out of the hospital to die at home, with just enough medically-trained support to allow comfort and dignity in death.

Now, as complementary medicine spreads, it is becoming more common to see nurses and physicians who do not intervene when patients choose to meditate in silence with their friends. As these changes are made, we open the gate to more interaction between the fields of medicine and Spiritism.

A Hopi elder gives sage advice about this time of change where many of our conventional institu-

Graphic displayed at Temple of Good Will depicting the four elements

32

tions, including medicine and religion, are adapting to new perspectives:

" There is a river flowing now very fast.

It is so great and swift, that there are those who will be afraid.

They will try to hold on to the shore, they will feel they are being torn apart and will suffer greatly.

Know that the river has its destination.

The elders say we must let go of the shore, push off into the middle of the river, keep our eyes open and our heads above the water.

And I say see who is there with you and celebrate.

At this time in history, we are to take nothing personally, least of all ourselves, for the moment that we do, our spiritual growth and journey come to a halt.

The time of the lone wolf is over.

Gather yourselves.

Banish the word struggle from your attitude and vocabulary.

All that we do now must be done in a sacred manner and in celebration.

We are the ones we have been waiting for."

Following are interviews with physicians I met in Abadiania who were willing to venture into the unknown, and pay a respectful visit to the world of spiritist healing. Because of these risk-takers, the gate which separates Spiritism and science can begin to be opened more easily for the rest of us.

All of the doctors I interviewed arrived in Abadiania reasonably skeptical and also willing to experience what the Casa had to offer. Each doctor had a different experience of the Casa de Dom Inácio, although all of them have had the opportunity to be close to the surgeries John of God performed. When I interviewed them, they were each in a process of re-evaluating how they want to practice medicine and how their experience at the Casa has changed them both personally and professionally. Reading their accounts may assist you in seeing how spiritist healing can be useful in conjunction with conventional medicine.

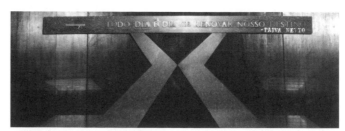

Altar at the Temple of Good Will

LEN SAPUTO, MD, DIRECTOR
HEALTH MEDICINE FORUM
WALNUT CREEK, CA

YEAR OF BIRTH: 1940
DUKE UNIVERSITY MEDICAL SCHOOL
BOARD CERTIFIED: INTERNAL MEDICINE

EMAIL: FORUM@HEALTHMEDICINE.ORG
WEBSITE: WWW.HEALTHMEDICINE.ORG

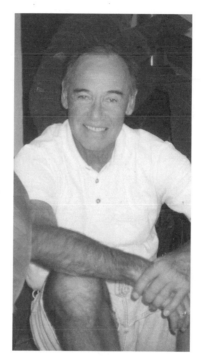

Saturday, August 18, 2001, a comfortably warm day, I sat with Dr. Len Saputo in the atrium of Pousada Dom Ingrid, a three minute walk from the Casa de Dom Inácio. In the background more than twenty indigo and white parakeets sang to each other as they flew around their seven by five foot cage. We heard an occasional scuffling of pots and pans in the nearby kitchen as breakfast dishes were washed up. Two resident dachshunds, who used the kitchen as their run, barked at passers by.

Dr. Saputo is the Director of *Health Medicine Forum*, developing a model for comprehensive clinical practice where conventional physicians cooperate with complementary health care practitioners in the same offices. With his wife, Vicki, a registered nurse, Dr. Saputo also co-hosts a radio program in the San Francisco Bay area, *Prescription for Health*. Listeners call in for advice and referrals regarding health care options. Dr. Saputo and Vicki are committed to assisting people in getting the best health care available. This commitment demands constant research and an ability to perceive a broad perspective.

Dr. Saputo began by saying that he finds himself at a time in his professional life where he is more and more willing to explore what is "out of the box," meaning, outside the beliefs that he was taught during his medical school training at Duke. He spoke with humor and compassion about his life as a physician, seriously considering options in health care he never would have considered before. He also spoke with the authority of one who takes pride in keeping current with the perspectives of conventional medicine:

"A health care system should both attend to the need to maintain perfect ability to function and attend to the need for meaningful purpose."

When two-thirds of all North Americans have a chronic disease and twenty-five percent of all Americans under eighteen have a chronic disease (e.g. asthma, cancer, ulcers, irritable bowel syndrome), we have an epidemic of chronic diseases that we don't know how to cure. The third leading cause of death now is our therapies, drugs, surgeries, bad advice, aka *iatrogenic disease*. [Definition of iatrogenic: induced unintentionally by the medical treatment of a physician.] The only thing that causes more death is heart disease and cancer. Not only are we ineffective with chronic conditions but we can't afford the cost of our health care system.

It's time for a wake-up call. What we do is actually less effective than we think, as measured by our own data, published in the Journal of American Medical Association and the New England Journal of Medicine! I want to encourage doctors to look at other paradigms which are more cost-effective and truly work.

I asked Dr. Saputo to share his definition of health and what he expects of health care systems:

Let's consider the way we usually look at health in the USA. Think of a scale with death at one end and perfect ability to function at the other. Symptoms are in the middle of the scale. The more symptoms you have the closer you are to death. Absence of symptoms we refer to as health. In the USA, people look for a body that works. We have a disease model rather than a health model. We look for absence of disease, absence of symptoms.

I prefer a model in which health refers to mind and spirit as well. Health care models from indigenous people work with the inseparability of body, mind, and spirit. In this model an essential indicator of health is that each person has a meaningful purpose in life and is manifesting that purpose.

A health care system should both attend to the need to maintain perfect ability to function and attend to the need for meaningful purpose.

When we, as individuals, know why we are here and what our contribution is, when we enjoy relationships and creative expression, then we can have true health.

You have to respect, love and appreciate your place in the universe first...accept that...love yourself this way...then your goal in life becomes to love and share. When you connect with others through loving intention, you can have real community.

"What is the aim of the incarnation of spirits? It is a necessity imposed on them by God, as the means of attaining perfection. For some of them it is an expiation; for others, a mission. In order to attain perfection, it is necessary for them to undergo all the vicissitudes of corporeal existence. It is the experience acquired by expiation that constitutes its usefulness. Incarnation has also another aim— that of fitting the spirit to perform his share in the work of creation; for which purpose he is made to assume a corporeal apparatus in harmony with the material state of each world into which he is sent, and by means of which he is enabled to accomplish the special work, in connection with that world, which has been appointed to him by the divine ordering. He is thus made to contribute his quota towards the general weal, while achieving his own advancement."

—from Kardec's "The Spirits' Book"

But, what medical students are trained to look at finding one's goal as an important part of attending to the health of patients? Most of what is transmitted to medical students these days is about medicating, intervening through our newest technology, monitoring and prolonging life even when the patient has no desire to live or no goal to live for. It is a rare physician who takes time to talk in depth to their patients about anything other than symptoms related to their illness.

Doctor's training is not based on connection with others. At Duke University, where I was trained, we looked at each person as a number and a diagnosis and prognosis. We didn't speak to a person— we spoke at the person with detached analysis. We didn't think of the mal-homeostasis we were contributing to. We were fixing...we weren't healing. Taking out a diseased gall-bladder, for example, removes a symptom but does not cure.

The people I trained with and most allopathic doctors today are immersed in a science based paradigm. What they can't understand doesn't exist. So, how can they speak about invisible spiritual worlds as real and look at another scientist straight in the face? If you don't understand it, it doesn't exist. Our stance vis a vis the world as physicians and health professionals was to be cold, analytical, detached, competitive, impersonal, separate, and adversarial.

What we do in training is learn to stay detached from our patients, be a scientist. It's a contradiction. We learn the opposite of what we should be doing. The job of the healer is to instill confidence and faith in each patient about who they truly are. Acknowledging them as spiritual beings is part of this job. If you are in a system where you don't have time to know yourself, or who the patient is and the patients don't know you—then none of this kind of deep healing can happen.

Now that we are learning more about physics, we are faced with some difficult truths about our science based paradigm. Actually, 50% of what we do is really science based. 1-15% of what is published is purely science based. 85-99% is projection. This means that there is a lot of illusion in what we have been calling science.

I want to drop the illusory aspect of being a "scientist" and participate more in what is really happening. But, being connected to myself, and with others is relatively new for me, so I have a lot to learn.

That's one reason that being here at the Casa de Dom Inácio has been very challenging for me, as well as inspiring. I think there is unlimited potential in the kind of healing which is offered here, but to receive it one must step into a more participatory point of view. To get what this is all about you have to get involved without being 'a know it all.'

A funny thing happened yesterday, my third and last day of participating in the activities of the Casa before leaving. I came down here to be of service to others, to witness the Entity doing surgery, to converse with a master from the point of view of another master, you know—exchange information, learn from each other. I envisioned sitting at a round table to see how we can work as a team. That's not how this place works. I was never invited to share my perspective with the Entity. After meeting him I was told to sit near him and just watch. I was put in the place of a new student.

After the morning session was over, I left the Entity's consulting room and I was walking through the assembly hall. Sebastian, João's secretary who has assisted him for over 20 years, was walking past me going the opposite direction. He was holding a bottle of water. Just as I walked by, Sebastian started to shake the bottle. But, there was no cap on the bottle so all the contents flew out and all over me. Not only had I just been placed in the position as a lowly new student, now I had water thrown on me and I had to walk around wet and disheveled in front of everyone. Sebastian just smiled pleasantly and walked on, indicating non-verbally, with an innocent shrug, that he had not realized that there was no lid on the top of the bottle.

I was at my wit's end for a few moments. I was thinking, 'Is there something wrong with me? Do they think I'm possessed with negative entities?' I felt so affronted, I considered packing up and leaving.

Now I have a new perspective. Maybe the entities of the Casa were responsible for my 'baptism' by Sebastian. After all, it was water that had been blessed by the entities which was showered all over me. And, the holy water bath helped me realize: 'Hey, I've only been here three days, and I think I am on the same level of knowledge that the Entity is? Who do I think I am? I have not earned a position here as having any authority. I only know a tiny bit about Spiritism. How can I possibly leave this place and think I can teach about it? *That* idea is much more destructive than constructive. I have so much to learn. I am certainly not in a position to tell the Entity what is right and what is not right.'

The Casa seems to be saying to me: 'Do you want to give us a try or not? If so, give up the arrogant attitude and humble yourself. Then you can see from new perspectives.'

Leaning forward, elbows on his knees, Dr. Saputo conversed with me as if I were a trusted companion. He was not protecting his authority or his position. He told me with conviction, very simply and clearly,

The seeds have been planted. I want to give it a try. I'll be back soon and stay for a longer period of time. Next time, I'll come as a student to learn. I'll study more about Spiritism first, be more receptive, and less arrogant.

In three days, I am impressed. Even though I didn't get to see any physical surgeries, I have come to recognize that there is a great deal of healing energy here. There is a potential huge upside and a negligible downside in being here. If I don't like what is happening I can stop—with no negative side effects. Right now, I don't know where the positive comes from. The assumption is it comes from João and the Entities. I suspect I will learn more about that when I spend more time here.

The process of learning more about myself and how I fit into the rest of humanity is clearly something very important that I can learn more about here. I feel like I already have more room for trust in myself and in the world of spirit—after only three days.

The Casa definitely has a role to play in redefining health and helping us to restructure health care delivery systems. This place is a model. Showing others an example of loving connection to each other and to spirits. The Casa offers a model of how

spiritual healing and prayer can work side by side. I see now that people can learn to connect intuitively to all that is in the world.

Personally, I want to connect and send energy in a vibratory way. Even though studying physics helped me see the rational side of this possibility by noticing that all things are vibrating at a certain rate. I had not been able to see that health professionals can empower vibrational shifts which are positive and transformative for patients. This was a revelation to me which I had never conceived of as real.

The Casa helps us experience more and understand more of the spiritual realms. Health care practitioners need to open more to spiritual realms because we learned nothing about the role of spirituality in medical school but we know that spiritual life contributes strongly to feelings of well-being, as well as healing. A real physician can only give what he or she owns. The more spiritually evolved the physician is, the more he/she can assist others in their own healing.

"Would you recommend a visit to the Casa to patients or doctors?," I asked. Dr. Saputo answered,

The Casa is an excellent place for anyone who wants to heal from disease or wants to do some spiritual growth. I also recommend the Casa to medical practitioners who want to move into a new paradigm.

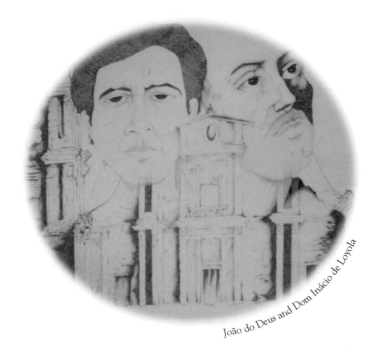

João do Deus and Dom Inácio de Loyola

ERICA ELLIOTT, M.D.
SANTA FE, NEW MEXICO
YEAR OF BIRTH: 1948

MA IN EDUCATION
BOARD CERTIFIED IN FAMILY PRACTICE AND
ENVIRONMENTAL MEDICINE

*Co-author: "Prescriptions for a Healthy House:
A Comprehensive Guide for Builders, Architects,
and Homeowners"*

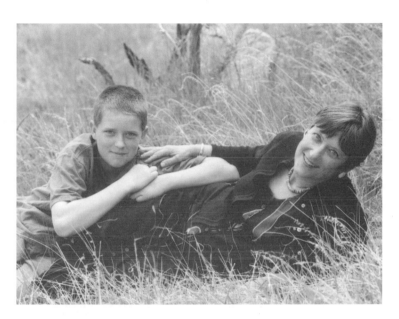

A former world class athlete and rock climber, she was the first American woman to climb Aconcagua, a 23,000 foot mountain in Argentina. She led an all-women's team to the top of Mt. McKinley in Alaska and has a peak named after her in Ecuador.

Dr. Elliott is a busy physician with a private practice in Santa Fe, New Mexico. She is also a single mother to her twelve year old son, Barrett, and president of her co-housing community. Dr. Elliott is well known for her work in Environmental Medicine. She has co-authored a book to help assist people in creating less toxic environments and has done extensive public speaking on the effects of chemicals on human health. She suffered from chemical sensitivities for ten years, after having worked in a toxic building.

Using altered states of consciousness in healing is not new for Dr. Elliott. As a young school teacher, before becoming a doctor, she lived with the Navajo Indians for two years at Canyon de Chelly in Arizona, and was an active participant in their peyote ceremonies, their portal to communication with spirits.

Dr. Elliott was well trained in conventional medicine. In her profession, paranormal experiences have been viewed with skepticism and often ridiculed. In order to excel in that paradigm, Dr. Elliott felt as if she needed to put a part of her soul in a little

"The Entity said, '...it's your turn now to get healed.'"

box on the shelf while she was in her training and for several years thereafter. But through her own illness, and because she has an irrepressibly curious mind, she began to veer away from mainstream dogma toward other forms of healing which were more congruent with her own beliefs and inner knowing, and which included healing energies. While she was aware of the ability to transmit and receive energy frequencies, she had had no direct experience with spirits.

Dr. Elliott was invited by a friend to go to Brazil to visit John of God in the Spring of 2001. She initially declined the invitation without having a thorough understanding of who John of God was. Shortly before her friend was to depart for Brazil, Dr. Elliott had a dream in which she saw herself taking a whole suitcase of photographs to João-in-Entity and having him help her with patients who were suffering with chronic, life-threatening illnesses. The next day she called her friend, and announced, "I'm going with you to Brazil." She later said, "Because of the dream, I felt like I was on a mission." This desire to help others served as a justification in her mind to make the trip and see the healer. Only later did she recognize that the trip was also necessary for her own personal healing.

When she actually met João-in-Entity in March, 2001, and went to hand him fifty-three photographs of her patients, the Entity said, "No, it's your turn now to get healed. We will work with them later." That same afternoon she began to take the herbs the Entity prescribed for her, deciding to focus on herself the first week and her patients the second week of her stay.

When Dr. Elliott went to the surgery room, as João-in-Entity had prescribed, she put her right hand over her heart, listened with closed eyes to the prayers and waited for the invisible surgery to begin.

At first, it seemed like nothing was happening. Then, I felt a current of energy coming into my right arm and into my heart. The space around my heart felt very warm, almost hot. The energy then traveled up to my left shoulder, down the arm and exited out my fingers and the palm of my hand. Just when I thought it was all over, another strong current of energy followed the same path. It was a strong and unmistakable sensation. After ten minutes, the session was over.

We were told to go back to our hotels and rest with our eyes closed. Being a high-energy person, I thought I'd never be able to stay in bed all day, not to mention keeping my eyes closed. Yet, on the way back to the hotel I found myself walking very slowly. I was deeply tired as though I had actually had a real surgery. At the hotel, I lay on the bed. As soon as I closed my eyes I felt the most blissful sensation of electric-like energy pouring into my head and swirling throughout my body. It felt like my whole body was being re-wired. After two hours my friend came into my room to check on me. She said that I looked different. She said it was especially noticeable in my eyes.

I felt a deep sense of peace. But I was also exhausted for no apparent reason. The fatigue was puzzling to me. I was told that when the entities are doing their healing work and the energy is moving around, it can leave people feeling very tired.

Over the following days Dr. Elliott had three crystal bed treatments, meditated and prayed in the current rooms. She felt a profound sense of peace.

During the two weeks of Dr. Elliott's visit to the Casa de Dom Inácio, she was invited to stand next to João-in-Entity three times and was asked to report to the audience, as well as live on videotape, what she saw the Entity doing in the visible surgeries. When the Entity scraped eyes with a paring knife, Dr. Elliott helped him by holding open the eyelids of the patient. Up close, she could see and feel that the patient showed no indication that he was experiencing pain and was not anaesthetized in the conventional sense. She also checked a patient after she watched the Entity cut into the man's abdomen, repairing a hernia. She reported that there was no evidence of the hernia after surgery.

When I asked Dr. Elliott what the Entity does in the procedure when he inserts a Kelly clamp up into the patient's nose, and rotates the instrument numerous times, she said, "It looks as if he reaches up the nose and into the brain as far as the pituitary gland. Under more 'normal' circumstances it would be extremely painful without anesthesia because there are so many nerve endings in this sensitive area in the nasal cavity and there would be the risk of causing brain damage, bleeding and infection... none of which happened."

The second week in Abadiania Dr. Elliott brought the Entity photos of her patients and her son, Barrett, who suffered with allergies and recurrent yeast infections. Almost a teen, he had a lifetime of low energy. The Entity accepted the photos and began his work on all these people through prayer.

Ten weeks after her visit to the Casa, Erica said that she can still access a profound peacefulness in herself, whenever she chooses to. She told me,

I can also sustain this feeling better than I used to. I can let go of anger and irritation quickly. Barrett tells me I'm a lot nicer. I am also less chemically sensitive and allergic. I can put gas in my car at the gas station without the strong reactions I used to have. I take my intuition more seriously. I am really curious to see how much more frequently I can make a correct diagnosis in difficult cases before I have even asked the patient for all the data. I still follow all the necessary procedures for evaluating the patient, but more and more often I can intuit the diagnosis well before I have the substantiating evidence to support my conclusions. I have renewed my daily meditation practice. Since returning from Brazil, I find I am more tuned in to energy, my own as well as that of those around me. I am recognizing that we each have our own way of perceiving extrasensory perceptions. Several clients have asked me to do energy work on them. They tell me they know I can help them this way.

For the purposes of researching spiritual healing and her own talents in this regard, Dr. Elliott decided to explore doing energy work with one of her patients, at the patient's request, shortly after the doctor's return from Brazil. I'll call the patient, Mary. Mary is a disabled physician who is so chemically sensitive that she would react to even minute amounts of pesticide residue brought into her home on the shoes of her friends. As a result, Mary had taken to living in her car. She had to use a respirator when she was in public places which contributed to her feelings of estrangement. She was suffering from isolation and felt very angry about her situation.

In their energy work sessions Mary lies on a massage table, set up in Dr. Elliott's office, which has been carefully furnished with non-toxic materials for those who are chemically sensitive. Dr. Elliott sits beside Mary in a chair. First, the doctor says a prayer, asking that spirits of healing guide her to help Mary in whatever way is right for Mary. (This is highly unusual for Dr. Elliott as she is not in the habit of praying with her patients.) Next, Dr. Elliott practices a form of laying on of hands, with the intention of drawing on universal spiritual energy to assist her. The sessions last an hour or more. After eight sessions, Mary appears to be improving, and continues to ask for more treatments.

"Healing has to do with becoming more whole within yourself, being more at peace with yourself, whatever your situation is in life. A cure is when the body has a complete remission of physical symptoms."

Several of Dr. Elliott's patients whose pictures were given to João-in-Entity have made remarkable progress in healing:

One of my patients was able to get off the ventilator in the Intensive Care Unit on the day that I brought her picture to the Entity. Another patient with a long history of suicidal depression felt joy for the first time in years, and is now off of all her medications because she continues to feel good. A third patient became significantly less chemically sensitive and had a big jump in the level of her energy. Several showed no changes, but the majority reported that they felt a sense of peace, along with some subtle shifts in their energy which they perceived as positive. Barrett's energy is now normal for a boy his age, his yeast problem has disappeared and his allergy symptoms are significantly better.

I asked Dr. Elliott what she tells people who ask her opinion about traveling to Brazil for healing work at the Casa.

I think approximately 10% of the people who come to the Casa have some immediate and long-lasting cure of their physical ailments. I tell my patients not to expect a dramatic cure. It's just not fair to set someone up with the expectation that they will be cured instantaneously. While there are dramatic successes which are awe-inspiring to watch and hear about, like people getting up out of their wheelchairs and walking again after years of being wheelchair bound, those who have these kinds of experiences are not in the majority. On the other hand, most of the people who go to see João experience some form of healing, if not a cure.

I make a point of differentiating between *healing* and *curing*. Healing has to do with becoming more whole within yourself, being more at peace with yourself, whatever your situation is in life. A cure is when the body has a complete remission of physical symptoms. If you are interested in becoming healed, the Casa is a wonderful place to go, where the majority of visitors experience a deepening peace and acceptance about their lives. Part of this healing has to do with connecting in various ways to the power of the spiritual forces which surround us.

The health professionals who are interested in going to the Casa are more likely to be ripe for a paradigm shift, if they haven't made one already. To leave your practice for a week or two to visit a sanctuary devoted to healing, and led by an unconscious medium, is very unusual in the world of physicians. You know you will be confronted with phenomena that cannot be grasped with the rational mind and you will have to grapple with how the experience at the Casa can be integrated into your life and into your practice of medicine. I would encourage any doctor ready to explore new perspectives to visit the Casa de Dom Inácio.

It became obvious to me that some people clearly have access to the spirit realm and can be especially useful in effecting healing in cooperation with spiritual realms. There is tremendous power in these interactions. How professionals come to terms with using this power in their practice and, in regard to their own personal growth, is quite an adventure. I look forward to the day when we have found a way to bring the best of our medical system together with what works in spiritual healing.

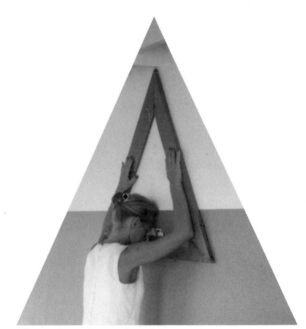

Woman praying by triangle at Casa

Frank Salvatore, MD.
Skylands Urology Group, P.A.
Sparta, NJ
Year of birth: 1961

Board Certified MD, specializing in Urology
Graduate of Georgetown Medical School

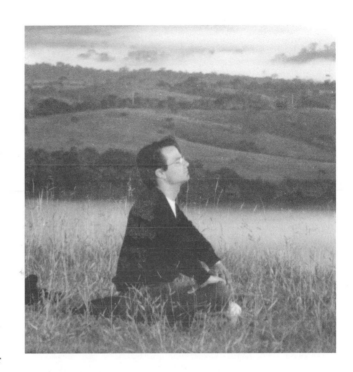

Dr. Salvatore went to the Casa de Dom Inácio for three days in April and three days in August, 2001. He wanted to continue his investigation of alternative forms of healing by watching Brazilian Spiritist healers. His medical school training had emphasized confronting physical problems through medical and pharmaceutical technology, and had overlooked the emotional and spiritual aspects of disease. Raised in a Catholic family and now a Hatha Yoga practitioner, Dr. Salvatore is open to new ways in which spiritual practices can effect health.

Like Dr. Herbert Benson, the Harvard Medical School professor who wrote *Timeless Healing: The Power and Biology of Belief*, Dr. Salvatore subscribes to the notion that belief in the means of healing is the most essential element for a patient in overcoming disease. He said,

Watching a Brazilian surrender to surgery by João-in-Entity is a striking example of the power of belief. The success João has had is a product of the purity of heart with which patients come to him. They believe wholeheartedly that he channels the power of God, that the Entity administers general anesthesia, and the entities around the Casa are wanting to assist in healing. Trust, or affirmative belief in a procedure, is the most potent indicator of success of the procedure. I think if someone goes to a Western trained surgeon or a Spiritist, like João, and does not believe that he will be cured by them, it will be nearly impossible for any healing process to work. It is not the procedure, per se, that does the healing—but the belief in the procedure that effects the healing.

"We need more understanding of the power of beliefs in healing."

Dr. Salvatore and I had the opportunity to converse over meals at the inn where our group stayed, and in several phone conversations on our return to the US. Currently in the midst of re-structuring the functions of his medical office, he was very open to looking at many different viewpoints about medical practice in general. Open-minded and bright, and clearly wanting to facilitate cross-cultural exchanges, Dr. Salvatore welcomed the opportunity to talk. I asked him for his ideas on how we might add to medical school training to help physicians understand more of the dynamics of healing as well as symptom control.

We need more understanding of the power of beliefs in healing. It's a new frontier for us. There are physicians who are pointing the way, for example, Deepak Chopra and Andrew Weil, but we need to increase the exposure which our students get to these innovators. Sometimes our indoctrinated beliefs get in the way: We have come to believe that patients *can not* get well unless they have surgery or drugs; but, sometimes patients can heal themselves without medical intervention from conventional medicine. Where a patient places his or her faith is a potent indicator for healing. Spontaneous remissions do happen. Spiritist healing alone can cure. Prayer can hasten healing.

As doctors we could strengthen our ability to witness our beliefs, and change those that are disempowering to ourselves or our patients. I'm not talking about positive thinking or affirmations which can be a superficial process. There are forms of one-pointed meditation where a person focuses on just one thought, and that thought penetrates every part of them. If that person focuses on the thought, 'I am healthy,' that individual will mobilize his whole system on an energetic, chemical and molecular level, to create health. It's powerful and very important in healing. Doctors could learn how to manage their minds more deliberately and teach those skills to their patients.

Energy dynamics also play a vital role in healing. In the current room at the Casa, where fifty to one hundred people meditate and pray together, their combined energy is focused like a vector, which empowers the work of the Entity in his healing with individuals. The combination of positive faith and positive energy is what makes the healing at the Casa work. These factors also create an environment which is healing for everyone. The patients, the healers, the volunteers, the children who sit by their parents who are meditating—everyone benefits. Everyone is receiving benefits from the spiritual energy generated by the group.

The spiritists can also help us understand more about an integrated approach to healing which includes working with energy and working with benevolent spirits.

Some doubters would ascribe the whole success of the Casa to the placebo effect, in other words, the belief in the healing creates the healing. My experience is that the work being done in the Spiritist Centers in Brazil transcends the placebo effect. There is an energy generated by people who are connecting with God which is very real and very effective in healing.

It's a big leap for us to seriously consider the role of faith, or any spiritual component, in healing as significantly positive. Not long ago, the Diagnostic and Statistical Manual of Mental Disease considered that talking to God or perceiving an angel was a symptom of psychosis. We preferred to perceive all that is invisible as unreal. This perspective replaced God, who is invisible, with psychologists and doctors. To turn around and say that close communion to spiritual realms and God is one of the most powerful contributors to creating health is a radical departure from where we have been.

Dressed for New York City, in his button-down blue shirt and kahkis, Dr. Salvatore relaxed into the backseat of the van as we sped down the highway from Abadiania towards the airport in Brasilia, on our way home. We asked the driver to stop so we could buy some coconuts from a vendor on the side of the road. The fruit was served up with a hole bored at the top and a straw to suck out the fresh milk. This treat was yet another new experience for Dr. Salvatore. For the first time in his life he had taken a day that week to go to a waterslide park for several hours—just for fun. "I just haven't had time to do this kind of thing before," he said, referring to the eighteen hour days he has been doing at work, six days a week. However intense his commitment to his practice, Dr. Salvatore is obviously a man who is willing to keep exploring. He recognizes that no one has the perfect magic bullet. He said:

I was impressed by the willingness of spiritist centers to work synergistically. I heard about the Entity recommending physical therapy, or chemotherapy, or radiation, or even psychotherapy along with continued prayer and faith in God. The Spiritists do not have a belief that a patient must only approach his/her illness from one direction. Instead there is a respect for the power and necessity of approaching problems from different avenues. Healing involves a process of working with the mind, the body and the soul. We are multi-dimensional. Each person is unique. Therefore, each person's healing process must be individ-

Illustration:
Angel sculpture from ceiling of
the National Cathedral in Brasilia, Brazil

ualized. Sometimes the Entity suggests, 'take the herbs, then decide with your doctor if you then want to do chemotherapy or radiation.' So, the Entity really empowers the individual to do what he or she feels is intuitively right—including listening to a physician's advice.

If the developed countries, like the US, want to be leaders in health care, we need to take a closer look at Spiritist healing. The Spiritist healers have had proven success treating illnesses, like cancer and AIDS, which we do not know how to treat effectively. The spiritists can also help us understand more about an integrated approach to healing which includes working with energy and working with benevolent spirits.

After all, it is part of our commitment as health care professionals to participate yearly in continuing education, and periodically open our work to the council of our peers. In this tradition we can go beyond national and cultural boundaries to investigate and recognize the power of healing practices in Brazil. It may help us to understand the universal nature of healing which applies to healing practices from every culture, not just Brazil. As we open up in this way, we will be in a better position to renew our medical school curriculum.

Finally, I asked Dr. Salvatore if there was anything more he would like to share about the significance of his trips to the Casa:

When I think back on my experience of being at the Casa de Dom Inácio I recall certain feelings. First, being in the presence of so many people, hundreds gathered together, all in need of healing, was humbling. Secondly, I felt a deepening faith in a Higher Power. I am sure that a spiritual force is involved in all that we do. I also feel it is important to do anything we can to open to this power. It will benefit us personally and professionally. Really, how can health practitioners deal with the vastness of human suffering? We must allow ourselves to be buoyed up by spiritual energy.

Would I recommend that others go to the Casa de Dom Inácio?

If you are a doctor and you believe that there is more to your work than drugs and physical procedures, then it will be a great benefit for you to experience the Casa de Dom Inácio. If you are a patient, and you feel that the Casa has something of value for you, then go and follow the inspiration which comes to you from your inner knowing.

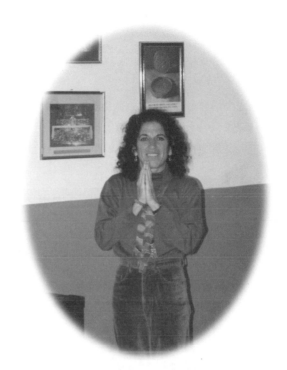

Nikki Schwartz, D.C.
Santa Fe, New Mexico
Year of birth: 1953

Graduate of Palmer West College of Chiropractic

In November, 2000, Dr. Schwartz came to the Casa de Dom Inácio for two weeks with high expectations. She wanted to witness the miracles she had read about and deepen her understanding of the spiritual roots of healing. Each day of her visit there were six hundred to two thousand people arriving by busloads early in the morning, waiting to see João de Deus. She told me her story:

When I met the Entity he prescribed herbs, suggested I have five crystal bed treatments and invisible surgery. I did all that the first week and I was actually a bit disappointed. There was nothing dramatic happening. I had no idea it was a preparation for the following week.

On Wednesday: the Entity asked me to come with him into the surgery room. There he approached a woman who was seated on a bench. He stood behind her, supported her head against his stomach, and proceeded to scrape her eyes with a paring knife, wiping the material he had scraped from her eyes onto her shirt. I was inches away from him. He looked at me, not the eyes of the woman, as he performed the surgery, giving me the clear message that another force was using his hands to do the surgery. It all seemed so natural and easy, I felt like I could do it if he had asked me to. The patient had had spiritual anesthesia and was experiencing no pain. At the end, the Entity said, 'She'll be fine.'

Next, the Entity went into the second current room, scanned the crowd meditating, singled out a man, and approached him. 'You have abdominal pain. Would you like to get rid of it?,' he inquired. The man, stunned that João had approached him, said, 'Yes, I have had constant pain for years in my abdomen.' He stopped short of asking, 'How did you know?' The Entity is known to see each person's blueprint, like an x-ray he takes in all the details of the health of each system and organ of the body.

The Entity asked the man to come forward and lean with his back against a volunteer. The man complied. Within seconds, the Entity palpated the man's abdomen, located a hernia, and made a three inch lateral incision. As he was making one incision with a knife, another incision appeared spontaneously just below it. There was no bleeding. João-in-Entity stuck his fingers into the man's gut by way of the incisions, moved his fingers around and then asked me if I wanted to check saying, 'There are already internal sutures.' I put my fingers into the open wound and could feel no evidence of a hernia. Soon after, the Entity stitched up the man's abdomen and he was taken to the recovery room to rest.

Days after, this man recounted that within one hour of the surgery the second incision had disappeared and he had felt very tired. He had rested. After four days he felt good, had only a faint scar, and no abdominal pain.

Dr. Schwartz was speaking to me by telephone. She thoughtfully selected words to tell her story, and at the same time, I felt as if our hearts were speaking a universal language which is beyond words. There was an ease and immediacy of understanding. Dr. Schwartz was not defending or protecting her professional role. I felt she was honestly and openly telling me about a part of her life story that had made a deep impression upon her. She continued:

The next surprise for me was an initiation. I was asked by the Entity to sit down in front of him, next to my friend, Eileen Karn, an acupuncturist. Catarina Pellegrino-Estrich was there to translate. It was made clear that this would be a ceremony to expand the healing energy of both Eileen and myself. The Entity reached for a needle and thread on the surgical tray. Immediately, I had a premonition, I thought, 'He's going to sew us together.' This is exactly what happened! Catarina invoked a prayer which helped me let go of my fear, 'Where there is God, there is no pain. Go to a higher place, sit in the flame of the heart of Jesus.' Then, the Entity pushed a needle into my hand through the web of my thumb. I could identify all the layers of tissue he went through, but felt no pain, only pressure. I had my eyes closed, but I knew he was also using the same thread and needle to go through the web of Eileen's thumb, too.

Suddenly I felt a tremendous influx of energy, as if I was a nuclear power plant. The horizontal bands of each of my chakras (energy centers of the body)

"I sensed I was surrounded by spiritual energies, as if I had been brought into a fold, a special gathering, and been acknowledged."

were vibrating. Emotionally, I felt bliss and happiness. After a short time, the Entity affirmed in prayer: 'You will work with this energy for the rest of your lives. You will work in joy for the rest of your lives.' I sensed I was surrounded by spiritual energies, as if I had been brought into a fold, a special gathering, and been acknowledged. Smiling lovingly, the Entity then cut the string, and invited us to sit in current.

I had an incredibly deep meditation. Most memorable was a voice which seemed to say to me over and over, 'What do you really want?' or 'What do you really need?' It was unusual for me to ask for things, and, frankly, scary to think that I might be getting assistance. But the message kept repeating itself very clearly. Each time I would say something like, 'I want my relationship to work out', this voice would say, 'Yes, fine and what else?' So, I continued, asking for things that I want: to fulfill God's purpose for me on this earth, to maintain this vast energy, to build a spa next to my home, and so on.

After the meditation a volunteer helped Eileen and me cut and pull the string out from our hands. It was about three feet long. The next day all that was left was a tiny bruise and a small hole, a reminder that the initiation really had happened.

Thursday Eileen and I were invited to come into the surgery room to examine the eyes of a Saudi Arabian Sheik. Before coming to the Casa this man had had laser surgery for a detached retina but the procedure had not relieved his problems.

The Sheik was lying down on a table. Eileen and I were asked to examine the eyes both before and after the Entity did energy work on them by placing his hands above the man's eyes, but not touching him. Each time energy work was done we noticed the eyes became more clear and there was less scarification. After the Entity did a few passes of this energy work, he asked a group of us to put our hands over the sheik to pass energy to him. I was at the patient's head, Eileen to my left, an Afro-American couple and a white American woman close by. The Entity put his hands over my head and energy started to move through me. Again, I felt like a nuclear power plant. This time the vibrations were so intense I had to move my hands and arms and body, as if I was dancing. It was totally out of character, out of my discipline, out of my professional persona, to be moving in this way.

The Entity then asked me, 'Tell me, how are your hands being used?'

I could barely think, much less talk. But somehow, I opened my mouth and said, 'My hands are being used as an instrument of the healing. My hands are being used like a scalpel cleaning out the film over his eyes which is the hate for his enemies, and giving it to God.'

As soon as I stopped talking, the energy started again. It was even bigger than it had been before. I was shaking and shaking, doing my best to give it to God. After a few minutes, my hands were moving in a different way, as if I had a feather fan which was now cleaning out the film over his eyes. The work was becoming more subtle.

Finally, the Entity put his hands on the eyes and forehead of the Sheik. He held him very strongly, really scrunching him tight, but the Sheik gave no indication that he was uncomfortable. Then, the Entity placed a sheet over the patient, covering his whole body including his face and eyes. It was a special covering embroidered with the six pointed star of David in the center. The Sheik was left to rest.

I felt we had addressed this man's eye problem, but more so, helped him heal the way he perceived the world, perhaps even the way he perceived others whom it was his habit to harshly judge. It was more about his soul than his body. The people who had been the instruments of his healing were three white North American women including a Jew and a gay Catholic, an Afro-American man and his wife, and an unconscious medium. Imagine, the Sheik had most

likely thought of these as the faces of his enemies, now they were clearly being his healers! I am sure this Sheik went back to his sphere of influence with a different viewpoint, a new way of looking at people whom his ancestors habitually dismissed.

Is this kind of surgery and drama necessary to create change and healing? No, I don't think so. The healing happens quietly, invisibly for the most part. I think the dramatic display is done as an outward expression of love for humans. We need to know that something is happening. It is hard for us to trust the forces that are invisible. We need demonstrations to validate the magnificent power of the inner planes. It seems as if we are imprisoned in concepts, separate and alone, in disbelief, when actually, we are not only being cared for, but all our wishes are being heard and attended to.

Ultimately, the force behind the Casa is God, or Love. It is huge. We need this vast energy to be stepped down so each person can connect with it at the level that is right for him or her. João in Entity serves that purpose. Like a transformer, he is a vehicle for divine energy to come to ordinary humans. He makes it accessible, as do the other entities who are available in the healing work of the center. As each one of us grows spiritually, we can align with more powerful energies and work as transformers, making God's energy of love more clearly available to others. The purpose of this life is to evolve spiritually. Physically, this means we can embody increasingly higher vibrations. But, each person has to go at the pace that is best for him or her. We can't do it en masse.

When I returned home I spent almost three months being as quiet as I could. I felt very introverted. I needed to rest. Now, six months later, I see how much my life has changed: Instead of seeing twenty-five to thirty-five people a day in my practice as I used to, I see one to five people a day. I do two to three hour sessions combining chiropractic work with massage in what I call "chiro-sage." I take more time to meditate and contemplate. I'm also considering new spiritual practices which will help me get even better at raising my vibration. I'm turning my home into a health spa/retreat center and looking forward to a lifestyle which is quieter.

I asked Dr. Schwartz to consider the success of the work at the Casa on two levels. First, is it successful in assisting individuals overcome their disabilities/illnesses? Second, is it successful in helping health professionals make a paradigm shift? She answered:

I saw miraculous results with individuals. I saw people who were cured of cancer, heart disease, and many other illnesses. I think João-in-Entity is generally more successful than our medical system.

Regarding the health professionals, I have less perspective. The people who come to the Casa select themselves. They are already unusual in that they are willing to travel to Brazil and expose themselves to someone who is an unconscious medium, doing healing work in Entity. There are many challenges in bringing this new paradigm back home to a culture that does not accept the presence of spirits.

The other challenge about importing this new paradigm is that the Casa is committed to attend to everyone without payment. Donations are accepted but no payment for services rendered. In North America our health care system is profit-based, just like the rest of our economy. How could anyone work hard and not accept payment? It's an anomaly. Even thinking about it makes people react strongly, as if their survival is at risk.

It would be interesting to follow-up, to see how much visiting health professionals can actually bring change into their practices and medical institutions once they get home. The work at the Casa just does not fit into the conventional paradigm. It's hard to introduce this new paradigm without being dismissed as irrational.

On the positive side—by visiting the Casa, a seed is planted. Those who have visited the Casa can hear a greater drumbeat. We see that there are lessons to be learned in each illness. Illness is not just an enemy to be destroyed on the material level. Illness presents us with a lesson that needs to be learned. It invites us to look at our lives more spiritually and less mechanically. If you destroy the symptoms of disease, it doesn't mean you have learned the lesson. In fact, you may have just avoided the lesson. Eventually, you will have to face it in another way.

Most of us are still enamored with materialism and used to fighting illness—as if the body was what life is all about. The perspective that our spiritual life is more important than our physical life has become interesting; but, how many people are really ready for this viewpoint, ready to make it real? When there is a critical mass of people embracing this new paradigm, i.e. committed to spiritual evolution, then we can create structural changes in the way we address health care and redefine health care systems.

As the invention of the microscope has revealed to us the world of the infinitely little, the existence of which was unsuspected by us, and as the telescope has revealed to us the myriad of worlds the existence of which we suspected just as little,—so the spirit-communications of the present day are revealing to us the existence of an invisible world that surrounds us on all sides, that is incessantly in contact with us, and that takes part, unknown to us, in everything we do. Yet in a short time, and the existence of that world, *which is awaiting every one of us*, will be as incontestable as is that of the microscopic world, and of the infinity of globes [realms] in space.

—From Kardec's "The Spirits' Book"

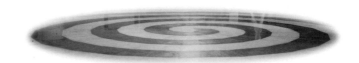

RICHARD SANDORE, MD
WADSWORTH, ILL.
YEAR OF BIRTH: 1961

BOARD CERTIFIED OB/GYN
MD DEGREE FROM UNIVERSITY OF ILLINOIS IN 1987
Currently a consultant and spiritual healer
WWW.SOARINGSPIRIT.COM

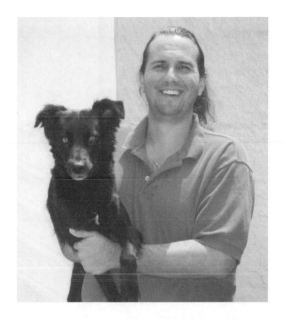

In the summer of 1992 Richard was sitting by his swimming pool at his country home, his porsche parked in the garage, his attractive wife by his side, his business partner totally committed to their successful private practice. In materialistic terms, he had made it. However, he felt despairing. He saw that thirty more years of this kind of life would not make him happy. In fact, he surmised he would feel that life had passed him by, if he stuck to the routines of being the physician he was trained to be.

Richard and I sat together on the tiled interior court of the inn where he was staying in Abadiania on September 18, 2001. Nine rooms on two levels in back of us were occupied by people who had come to visit the Casa de Dom Inácio with Richard as their guide. Facing us was the apartment of Martin and his family. Martin, who owns the Pousada, is also head of the team of translators at the Casa and takes care of the special needs of people who come from all around the world to consult with João. Just outside the courtyard door was third world Brazil: dry, poor, simple, trafficked with horse-drawn carts, occasional cars, and adults bicycling to work. Two stray mongrels, one black, the other white, had adopted Richard and lay at his feet.

It was a critical moment when I realized that summer day that I still didn't know who I was, where I came from, what I was doing on earth and where I was going. I had to find a way to answer these questions as soon as possible.

Within six months I turned my life around. I started studying shamanic tradition from numerous heal-

"I have also developed a whole different standard on which to judge healing."

ers, especially those connected to South America. In June, 1998, I was working for a non-profit organization bringing medical care to an area of the Andes mountains, so I could simultaneously work with healers in Peru. That was the year I found out about João de Deus and spent a week at the Casa de Dom Inácio. A year later I brought seventeen people here to visit. This week, my seventh trip here, I am purchasing a home in Abadiania.

My main interest here is to develop a relationship to the entities associated with the Casa de Dom Inácio. I have not been working on any personal physical problems. I have been asking questions about my path in life and the answers come to me when I am "in current." I have acquired much more confidence and faith in my work.

I have also developed a whole different standard on which to judge healing. In medical school and in private practice I judged my success as a doctor on whether a disease process would go away. If the person was symptom free, then I felt like I was a success. If the patient still suffered from symptoms, I felt like I was a failure. Now I feel that my success as a healer depends on whether the patient feels more whole and more at peace. I want to hear from them that they perceive their world as being all right

as it is. I want them to feel that they are perfect just the way they are. This may include accepting the illness they have or being symptom-free. Reaching this state of mind is the kind of health I am helping my clients achieve.

I asked Richard, "How is your practice as a healer different from your practice as a physician?"

Relaxing back into his white molded plastic chair, he replied,

Using my intuition has become central to my work. I did not learn this skill in medical school, in fact, we were not taught to honor our intuition in school or residency. We were also not taught to honor the individuals who were our patients, and to consider their values. Now, I use my intuition to feel the nature of the person in front of me. I can be more empathic as a result. This enhances our connection. The patient feels heard and respected and, as a result, he or she feels safe to reveal more of the essence of the problem. I also feel more at ease asking blunt questions. Our relationship is founded more on trust and faith in ourselves as two individuals, rather than the patient abandoning him or herself and just placing faith in the doctor.

I remember one woman who was in the final stages of cancer when she came to me. Her husband was beside himself with worry. He didn't want to lose her. I asked the woman what she wanted. She told me she was ready to die, that she was satisfied with her life and could leave it behind. She didn't have a problem with dying. Most doctors are trained to do everything they can to save the patient, but, in this case, I felt it was important to let the woman die peacefully and turn my attention to her husband. He was really the one with the problem. He was suffering far more than his wife, in this case.

Medicine in its inception was recognized as an art. People are multi-faceted. Our values and our perspectives are in flux. Our doctors need to be attentive to who the patient is at any given moment, and not treat the patient as a disease. People who are ill or in pain are on a healing journey. The journey pushes their comfort zones and makes them develop new perspectives. They need allies on the journey. Our conventional practice of medicine is being reduced to reading computer programs, where you write in your symptoms and the program matches them with a disease and treatment program. There is no human connection in this. There is no possibility for empathy, compassion and the most healing force of all: love.

As Richard and I settled into the interview, I began appreciating his steady warmth and humanness. At forty, Richard retained a youthfulness, accentuated by informal clothes, a five inch ponytail, and a ready smile. As we sat down with the tape-recorder on, I was feeling relieved to have a distraction from the disastrous events of the last week. Terrorists had used airplanes as missiles to destroy the World Trade Center and a portion of the Pentagon. Those of us in Brazil were wondering when the airports would open again for international travel and if our country would soon be at war. Although we began by sharing our deep concerns for the world, Richard gracefully shifted to the present moment — enjoying the interview and what was positive about 'now.'

I asked Richard to consider what physicians might learn by traveling to the Casa:

Physicians can learn many things by coming to Abadiania and participating in the activities of the Casa. First, nothing is impossible. Therefore, we have to put aside our statistics and not give someone a prognosis which has them believe they will soon be dead. The mind is powerful. If someone believes they will soon die, they can persuade the mind to create that as a reality. The limits we put on ourselves

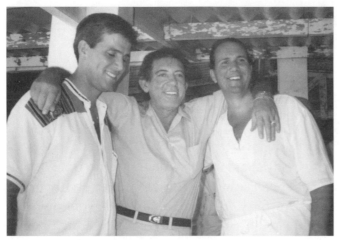
Martin, João and Richard

or our patients are determining factors in their ability to heal. Our attitudes and our beliefs about our patients may bring them to better health or erode what health they have.

I am learning more and more that the patient knows what he or she wants and needs. Sometimes, that person needs to sit quietly and get in touch with his or her truth. It may not be contained in any book. But, it is within them. I have come to respect this as the most important part of health. Every person's journey is individual and unique and should be respected as such.

When I visit the Casa, I am always impressed by the compassion and understanding that is offered people as individuals. Also, people have very different experiences when they sit in current—or talk to the Entity. Physicians learn how inappropriate it is to treat patients as holders of a specific illness, with a statistically determined outcome. We learn to open up our ability to treat people as individuals on unique journeys.

I have noticed that doctors can not open to this level of connection with their patients until they open to this level of connection with their own journey within themselves. They need to be willing to give up the role of being a God on a pedestal. They need to learn more skills in connecting to people, respecting others, having faith in others, honoring others. They need to learn more about trusting themselves.

Richard is so enthusiastic about the value of visiting the Casa de Dom Inácio, I asked him if he suggested coming here to everyone who might be interested. He replied,

I like to invite people to come. Then, I suggest they follow their intuition. They know in themselves if there is something at the Casa which will be of value to them on their own journey.

99% of the people I have brought here feel it has been a positive experience. The only person who has been displeased was a doctor who was not open to giving up his perspective on health and healing. He was not interested in being at peace, or facing his Creator. I feel that there is something here for everyone, providing someone is open and willing to learn something new, to learn new ways of seeing and being.

ANNEKE S. VISSER
THE NETHERLANDS

YEAR OF BIRTH: 1935
EMAIL: ANNEKESARAH@YAHOO.COM

DOCTOR OF HOMEOPATHY AND NATUROPATHY
CERTIFIED BY ACADEMY OF NATURAL MEDICINES
THE NETHERLANDS
Advanced studies in Chiropractic
and Applied Kinesiology at the School of Osteopathy,
London, England

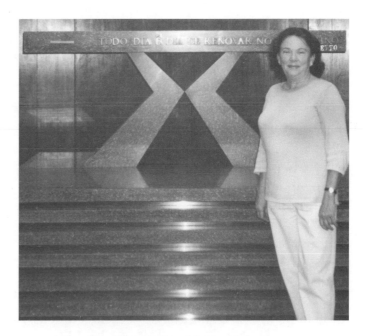

Anneke and I walked from our Inn to the garden of the Casa de Dom Inácio for our interview, September 9, 2001. In keeping with the ease with which everyone becomes equal at the Casa, Anneke would not allow me to call her Dr. Visser, but preferred "Anneke."

An attractive woman, in her bright pink top, decorated with cats of varied colors, and her elegant black slacks, she could have fit into a resort anywhere in the world. Born in Holland, she had, in fact, traveled and lived in many different countries, including staying seven years in Wisconsin, studying and teaching the Course in Miracles, the channeled teachings of Jesus.

Anneke attended a United Nations congress of religious leaders in the summer of 2000, followed by a congress of the world's political leaders. She came to Brazil in late July, 2001. This was when she realized that Brazil is the one of the only cultures on the planet which is one with the world of spirits. This unity is one of Brazil's gifts to the world.

Anneke has been in private practice as a homeopath since 1980. Soon thereafter she was invited to be a consultant to physicians wanting to use homeopathy and naturopathy to complement their more conventional medical treatment procedures. Acupuncturists, oncologists, internists, and dermatologists seek her advice on their most difficult patients.

Since the age of six, Anneke had experiences with her own clairvoyance and clairsentience. She laughed heartily when she admitted the gifts went away when she was fifteen years old and she kept falling in love with her sisters' friends. The psi abilities returned when she was living in East-Africa with her husband, and doing volunteer work at a hospital. She began to feel the suffering of the patients without rational knowledge of what was wrong with them. This inspired her to develop her gifts as a doctor. Clearly devoted to understanding the root of healing and bringing that to others, Anneke is looking forward to opening her own health center in Europe in the near future. She is considering patterning this new center after the Casa de Dom Inácio.

I asked her why she came to Abadiania and if she would recommend it to others:

I wanted to see how John of God works and to see if I could connect with the entities. I also wanted to get rid of a tropical parasite, Bilhartzia, which I have had for thirty years. Conventional medicine has no effective cure for this condition. My husband died of it fifteen years ago.

Since I have been here, almost two months, I feel more energetic. The functioning of my digestive and circulatory systems has improved. I feel like my organs are becoming healthier. When I used to sit to meditate I was agitated, and my thoughts were chaotic and unrelated. Now, when I sit I can just be, or I can think about what I want to think about in an organized way. My nervous system is quieter. The transformation, or resurrection of the spirit, is a slow process, but that is OK. I can take the time to do it. In fact, I want to take the time. You have to change your thought patterns to make yourself healthy. Every emotion, every thought triggers your chakras and your endocrine system in particular ways. When you open your heart, and stop perceiving yourself as a victim, you can create a physical resurrection. It is like being born again in this same lifetime. The Casa de Dom Inácio is a very special place and I am continuing to learn more about healing every day.

The entities who attend patients here are very evolved. They do not have emotional reactions. They have no need to be right, to be arrogant, to assert their self-importance. They are beyond that. They simply are available to be of service to those who sincerely ask for help. They have evolved past the point of needing to reincarnate. They have learned the lessons of life on earth. They have become *a brotherhood of truth and love*.

"The cure here is rarely instantaneous. Instead it is a kind of resurrection, a being born into a new relationship with your spirit and your body."

I find that my clairvoyance is becoming stronger as I stay here and continue to meditate, study, and experience the love of this place. I can sense the presence of entities and discern one from the other. This began happening when I sat in the second current room near the Entity when he was doing his work. But, I think the understanding that Brazilians have, that we are all deeply connected to spirits on the other side, and that some of these spirits can help us, is one of the most powerful forces of change I have seen here. Those who come from the so-called developed nations can experience that we are not separate from spiritual realms or spiritual qualities.

I see the volunteers at the Casa always looking to see how they can help each person be more comfortable. They are helping us to experience the tremendous love, the infinite love, which is here for us if we are open to experience it. The love is both earthly, where people treat each other with kindness, and unearthly, where people are healed by entities from spiritual domains. Many people report feeling a warm glow of happiness around the presence of entities. It brings new life to what Christ taught, to treat each person as your brother.

You don't have to be Catholic or even Christian to feel at home here. I am Rosicrucian. I enjoy saying the Lord's prayer with everyone. I appreciate seeing people from all faiths here. I also appreciate the fact that I see only one cross. I've never liked the vision of Christ, the martyr, suffering on the cross. For me, Christ is a positive and life-affirming presence, a resurrected teacher; there is no death—we only lay down our physical bodies. Here in the Casa it is a fact, a fact you can experience every moment.

The cure here is rarely instantaneous. Instead it is a kind of resurrection, a being born into a new relationship with your spirit and your body. If you are here for a while, and sincerely continue the work through continued prayer and meditation, being responsible for your thoughts and actions, you identify yourself more as the spirit you are, and use your body to do the work your spirit came into this life to complete. I think of illness as being a great awakener for some people as it takes them to ask themselves, 'Why am I here on earth?' and 'Why did I come into this world of pain and misery to eventually die? Why does this cycle of birth and death happen over and over again?'

Many people have to become more self-responsible and clear. We are here to not only clear our own karmic patterns, but help clear the karma of mankind. Humans have done terrible things to each other for thousands of years. Think of the pogroms of World War II where millions of Jews were tortured and killed. Most importantly, we have to forgive ourselves for this ignorant and violent behavior, and then restore ourselves by living a more compassionate life.

I originally came here for two weeks on a tour, then I decided I had to stay longer. This is not a place to be a tourist. You have to respect the fact that being here represents entering a process. It is not appropriate to see the Entity on Friday, and then sit in a car and go touring for three hours—just because you like to see waterfalls. You have to humble yourself, simplify your life, and take quiet time to yourself in gratitude for the opportunity of being here in this powerful spot where entities are available to you. It takes discipline to continue the work but the results are well worth it. You are healing your heart and mind, not just your body. You come to see, with new eyes, that everyone is your brother. I can understand why people come here for months, even years, at a time.

I recommend this place to anyone who wants to truly heal the split between their body and their spirit. You need to have some belief that beneficent entities exist who want to help you. After that, be willing to work on yourself. Then, relax and let the process unfold.

We walked back to our Pousada (inn) together. I had the feeling that we had been friends for lifetimes.

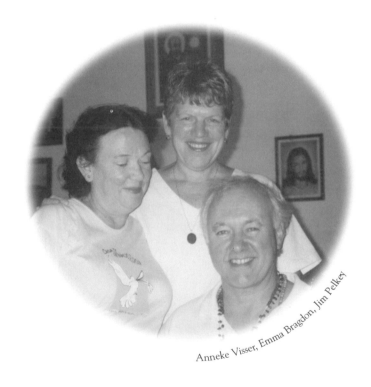

Anneke Visser, Emma Bragdon, Jim Pelkey

63

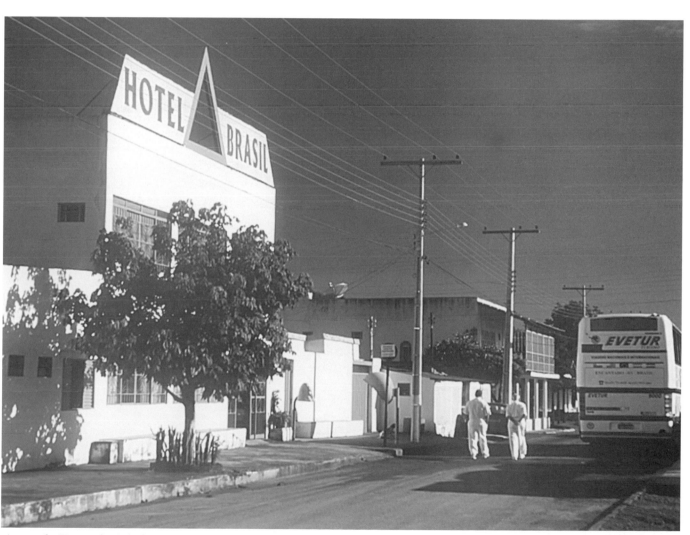

Avenida Frontal, Adadiania: toward the Casa

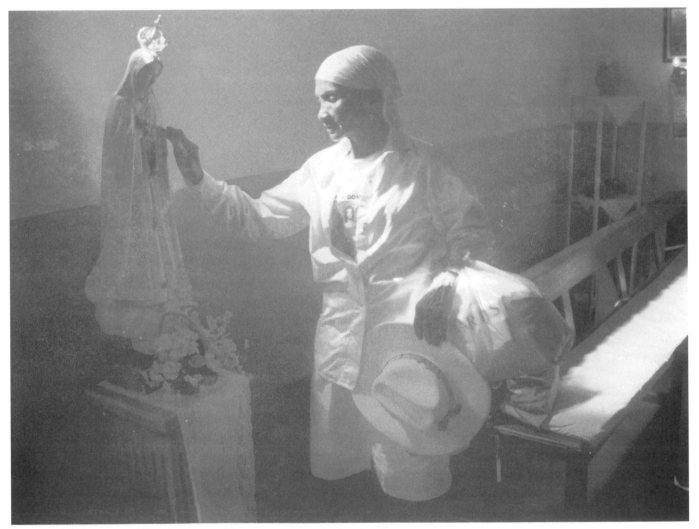

Brazilian medium after a session of morning Current at the Casa.

PART FOUR: PARTNERS IN CREATING HEALTH

I was in the Entity's room meditating when it was announced that we could open our eyes to watch an operation. Fome, a Brazilian woman, in her thirties, from Abadiania, stood facing in my direction, about six feet in front of me. Her shirt was pulled up, the waist of her pants loosened around her hips to expose her belly. Even though her features were quite plain, she looked like the Madonna—completely peaceful and relaxed, eyes wide open, steadily beaming an extraordinary love and compassion.

I watched the Entity use a surgical knife to make a four inch incision into Fome's lower abdomen. A bit of blood wept around the opening. Fome observed with some interest—and not a flicker of fear or a wince of pain. The Entity stuck three fingers into the incision, moved them around for a few seconds, and extracted a small mass. He rolled it between his fingers studying it, discarded it, then cleaned his hands in water and asked a volunteer to suture the wound. Fome continued to stand without support, patiently waiting as the volunteer slowly found needle and thread, knelt in front of her, and sewed the edges of the cut together.

Time seemed to disappear into the vastness of Fome's faith. She was the epitome of a steady belief that she was in the right place at the right time—receiving something real, something good. Beneficent spirits working through the Entity was what the world had to offer her as a way to take care of the tumor growing in her uterus. There was no doubt in her mind, and no hesitation in her body.

I hope I never forget the sight of Fome's certainty and peace. This is what is possible when spiritual knowing completely infuses the physical body: a powerful spiritual alliance.

Spiritist healing has often been dismissed as simply "faith healing" or the "placebo effect." Substantial research has demonstrated the power of our beliefs: when a person believes he or she will be healed, the belief can change the chemistry of the body and *create* the healing. Conversely, when a person believes she will die, she can die, even if there is no apparent 'cause of death.' Faith healing occurs when one places such faith in the power of a healer that healing occurs in the presence of that person. If a person places total faith in a pill, believing that the effects of the pill will cure or relieve

"...placebo is always present in spiritist healing, as it is in all medical practices, to one degree or another."

symptoms, the pill will more than likely perform the desired task. This is the "placebo effect."

Our knowledge of the placebo effect is used in diverse ways. Sometimes it is used to dismiss the value of some therapy or procedure, for example, "there is nothing of intrinsic value there, it's *only* placebo." Sometimes knowledge of placebo is applied proactively — to harness energy to implement healing through belief management. Master hypnotherapists have developed this skill. Milton Erickson acquired a reputation for being able to heal someone from a long-standing phobia within minutes, simply by changing the patient's viewpoint in a dramatic way. Dr. Frank Salvatore, interviewed in Part Three, said:

As doctors we could strengthen our ability to witness our beliefs. We can learn to change those that are disempowering to ourselves or our patients. I'm not talking about positive thinking or affirmations which can be a superficial process. There are forms of one-pointed meditation where a person focuses on just one thought and that thought penetrates every part of them. If that person focuses on the thought, 'I am healthy,' that individual will mobilize his whole system on an energetic, chemical and molecular level, to create health. It's powerful and very impor-tant in healing. Doctors could learn how to manage their minds more deliberately and teach that skill to their patients.

Mark Woodhouse, the author of "Paradigm Wars," suggests that the efficacy of all our medical practices is the history of the placebo effect, i.e. managing beliefs. As time and technology move on, we *believe* in one method of cure, then the next. It is our *belief* in our doctors and their cures that profoundly impacts the degree to which we are cured, not simply the advances in technology or medicine. Thus, doctors are consciously or sub-consciously using the placebo effect while attending to their patients.

From this vantage point one might consider that all that goes on at the Casa de Dom Inácio is faith healing and the placebo effect. Here is a way we can dismiss the work of spiritist healing, consider it illusion, and return to our indoctrinated beliefs of what is "real." *However, in this case, we lose a valuable opportunity. We run the risk of denying the possible reality of spirits and healing through the intentional direction of energy.*

A piece of Ryan Elliot's film, "The Healing Ministry of John of God," shows a woman being

A degree of placebo effect ————————> creates healing

A degree of placebo effect ————————> creates bio/physical change/relieves symptoms

operated on by João-in-Entity. After making the incision in her back with a surgical knife, it took fifteen minutes for the Entity to clip, pull, and tease out the lemon size lipoma (fatty tumor) from around her spine and connective tissue. The patient's surgeon, in the USA, had not been willing to perform the surgery for fear that it would irreversibly damage his patient's spinal cord. The Entity was able to complete the surgery successfully. The patient was able to sit peacefully for the surgery with the aid of spiritual anesthesia. She had no medicine for local or general anesthesia, only the "spiritual anesthesia." This can not be ascribed solely to the "placebo effect." Perhaps benevolent spirits at the Casa de Dom Inácio do impact lives by giving patients anesthesia, directing the surgeon's knife, minimizing blood flow, and accelerating healing.

Rather than dismiss spiritist healing, we might consider that placebo is always present in spiritist healing, as it is in all medical practices, *to one degree or another*. Imagine a person who is sick. Seeking relief, he or she goes to a spiritist healer or to a conventional doctor. In the case of consulting with a spiritist, it may be simply the placebo which effects the healing; or, some degree of placebo, or solely the action of spirits.

In the case of consulting with a conventional physician it may simply be placebo which effects the healing; or, some degree of placebo, or solely the action of chemical or surgical intervention, or physical manipulation, as in setting bones. It is a common joke that some people become cured of an illness simply by going to the doctor's office. Has it ever happened to you? "Sorry doctor, I was coughing all night and somehow right this minute, seeing you, all the symptoms are gone." Some people have healed from illness when they have an operation which opens the abdomen and the surgeon removes nothing, then sutures the wound.

Our trust, or belief, in the method of healing is an essential part of the process...no matter what healer or health care practitioner we consult. However, our trust in the healer is not the only element necessary...in fact, some healing seems to take place in spite of a person's lack of belief. Spiritist healing works on skeptics who do not believe in it as well as those who do. (This should be a subject of further study. The results would assist us to better understand the power of spiritist healing and the effects of placebo.)

Those who would dismiss healers such as João de Deus as simply creating trances, or hypnotizing their subjects to create the placebo effect, should also consider this: healers achieve demonstrable results on non-human subjects. Human energy has been directed to mice, enzymes, yeasts, and the surface tension of water, in varieties of laboratory tests.[1] As a result of directing energy from the body to a non-human organism, the organism changes it's molecular structure in measurable ways. None of these organisms have belief systems so how can the changes they make be ascribed to placebo?

In the fight against degenerative diseases, spiritual healing is still on the sidelines, often relegated to the bench, overlooked as a valuable player, and cast in the role of "last resort." When we consider that we have helpers in spiritual realms who want to be of assistance, and we invite them in to help us, our job with health care may become much easier. Kardec wrote:

"Spirits are everywhere; the infinitudes of space are peopled with them in infinite numbers. Unperceived by you, they are incessantly beside you, observing and acting upon you; for spirits are one of the powers of Nature, and are the instruments employed by God for the accomplishment of His providential designs. But all spirits do not go everywhere; there are regions of which the entrance is interdicted to those who are less advanced."
—from Kardec's "The Spirits' Book"

If help is there, shouldn't we make use of it?

Following are Interviews with several people who decided to come to the Casa de Dom Inácio as part of their healing process. These people are truly participants in their own healing, as they had to take considerable initiative. One had to fly across the Pacific Ocean even though he had been told he would probably die on the trip. One decided to risk his last ounce of energy standing in line for hours to see João de Deus. Most chose not to tell their physicians what they were doing. For better or for worse, they went beyond the conventional norms, because they wanted to explore another avenue in healing. These people have courage. They also have some degree of faith in the possibility that spirits can help us in our healing.

The medium João said:

"For those who believe, no words are necessary. For those who do not believe, no words are possible."

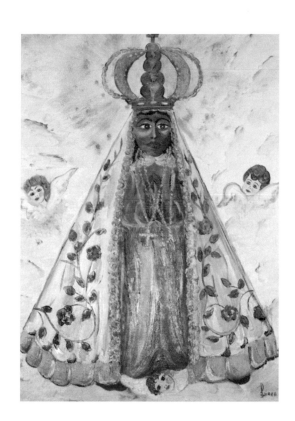

CHRISTOPHER SHEPPARD
ENGLAND
YEAR OF BIRTH: 1952
Film Producer

In November, 1999, Christopher was diagnosed — out of the blue — with rectal cancer. He is now healthy again. The tumour has completely disappeared, without needing the surgery that the doctors had urged upon him. Christopher said,

I intuitively believed the causes of my illness were to be found within my own life and that I hadn't gotten sick because of an accident of fate or genetics or bad luck; I believed that there would be causes within my own life that I could understand and unravel and then put straight. In the case of having a tumour, as I did, it seemed common sense that my body had made it and that therefore my body could un-make it.

This point of view got reinforced as I went along, both through what I experienced myself and through the books I started to read (foremost among these were *Getting Well Again* by Carl Simonton and *Love, Medicine and Miracles* by Bernie Siegel, both written by doctors whose first-hand clinical experience forced

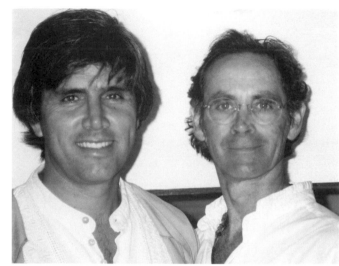

Martin Mosquera and Christopher Sheppard

them to change their views on healing.) I became absolutely convinced that body and mind are intimately linked when it comes to sickness and health, and that your mind can be your most powerful tool in healing from cancer.

Christopher decided to trust his judgment and intuition in finding his own way through cancer. He also sought advice from medically astute friends to help him choose from the plethora of healing options available to him. Ultimately, he drew from the recommendations he got from acknowledged leaders in various fields of both allopathic and complementary medicine, piecing together a protocol which involved physical, emotional, and spiritual approaches. Essential physical approaches included diet, immuno-therapy, acupuncture, osteopathy, homeopathy and radiotherapy (see glossary.) He lived mainly on fresh organic juices, brown rice and vegetables. Emotional healing included support groups, a form of emotionally-expressive therapy, and hypnotherapy. Essential spiritual approaches were his visits to the Casa de Dom Inácio in Abadiania and Tibetan Buddhist meditation.

His is not a case of an instant miracle at the Casa. However, it is an inspired case of documented cure—in which the Casa played a central role. The patient was decidedly active in treatment, and was sustained by a loving partner and friends. His story demonstrates how healing of the spirit must be integrated into every aspect of life: physical, emotional and spiritual. When I met Christopher in December, 2001, he was celebrating his one year anniversary of being told by medium, João, that his healing was complete. He had come back to Abadiania to express his gratitude and, again, enjoy this spiritual sanctuary.

Following are excerpts from an interview Christopher did with his partner, Sally. The full interview, exploring all of his story with cancer, is accessible on www.christopher-sheppard.com. The site includes resources for the alternative cancer treatments Christopher used. I highlight the spiritual aspects of his treatment to provide another viewpoint on how visiting the Casa de Dom Inácio can effect healing.

CHRISTOPHER: The biggest and the single most radical step that I took was to pursue spiritual healing. Three weeks after my diagnosis I was on a plane to Brazil to see João de Deus. I stayed for six weeks.

This was a very radical choice because spiritual healing was not something I'd ever been involved in, not something I knew very much about. It emerged as a choice because I was aware that I needed to do something extreme. In deciding not to have surgery, the stakes were raised considerably, and I was getting a lot of messages from those around me — therapists, healers, family and friends — that I was in a precarious position, and that strong action was called for.

Q: In what sense was this a spiritual journey?

CHRISTOPHER: It started by my accepting that the cancer I had was more than just a physical illness: it was an energetic thing too, an expression of an emotional and spiritual malaise. In addressing that malaise and trying to heal it, I came to feel that it was possi-

"...there was a very complex set of causes within my way of living and my way of being, which lay deeply at the source of my illness and which I had to address."

ble for me to call upon a source of energy outside myself, that for want of a better word I'd have to call "divine" energy. I started to believe that it was possible to access a source of healing power that was greater than me, although it still relied on me as the ultimate instrument of my own healing.

Q: This work in Brazil proved to be a central part of your healing process?

CHRISTOPHER: It absolutely clicked with my feeling that the task I was facing was that of trying to heal my whole being. This corresponded with my more reasoned judgement in deciding not to have surgery: the belief that the surgery might remove the physical symptoms but would do nothing about correcting the causes (which also seemed to go some way to explaining the conventional wisdom that following any surgery for cancer there is the threat of spread or recurrence: the symptoms may have been temporarily removed but the underlying causes may remain). Going to Brazil on this spiritual journey opened up the space for me to start to understand that there was a very complex set of causes within my way of living and my way of being, which lay deeply at the source of my illness and which I had to address.

I realised that for years I had been neglecting myself as a spiritual being; and was in denial about some difficult realities in my life. I was deceiving myself and those around me about what was really going on inside me. Put bluntly, without realising it I had become a liar. This was compounded by the sudden death of my mother (six months before the diagnosis) coming in the middle of enormous difficulties at work. My life was in a mess—a mess which I was neither fully aware of nor able to face up to. All this resulted in a split within me; a psychic, spiritual and emotional split that was both an expression of, and in some ways also a cause of, the splitting at the deepest cellular level in my body. Cancer cells were splitting away from normal, healthy cells to the point where one type of cell could not recognise another.

Q: In that sense the illness seemed like a metaphor for what was happening in your life, manifesting in your body?

CHRISTOPHER: Yes. And the message that this gave to me was that the real work, the deepest healing work that needed to be done, was both spiritual and emotional. (This seemed to correspond with what I learned later about cutting-edge research in molecular biology showing that individual cells have an emotional memory which can make them "sick." Dr. Deepak Chopra makes a similar argument in his book *Quantum Healing*. And scientist Candace Pert explains it in her book *Molecules of Emotion.*)

Q: How did you do this spiritual and emotional work?

CHRISTOPHER: Well, the first thing to say is that my life became a rollercoaster. This was not the cool, calculated process that an account like this may make it seem. Terror and rage and grief all played their part, and my life was lived continually at the edge, often in a tempest of uncertainty and conflict with those around me. I was afraid of dying - and there were those around me whose private view was that I would die. And at times the tearful, sometimes heartbreaking repercussions of all the truth-telling in my personal life merged inseparably with the fight for life. But again and again these dramatic struggles returned me to the spiritual and emotional work which I firmly believed was at the heart of my healing.

The spiritual work I did in two ways. First, using the opportunity that was provided by the Casa de Dom Inácio in Brazil. Although it calls itself a healing center, it is a cross between a sort of clinic and a church, where two important things happen. The "shop window" of the place, the sensational side of it, is the demonstration of extraordinary, almost paranormal healing phenomena, where actual surgical operations are undertaken by the Entity without anaesthetic or proper instruments. Behind this is the belief, that is central to the work there, that you must heal the energy (or the "soul" or the "spirit") before you can heal the body, and that a lot of this healing work is done through meditation and prayer. One important function of the Casa is to provide a context for intensifying a force field of belief, of faith, and of concentration among the people there, which magnifies the possibilities of using healing energy, whether it's "divine" or however one describes it.

The other key thing about the Casa is the emphasis that it puts on each individual taking responsibility for his or her own healing. A favourite refrain of the spirit medium when people come and ask to be healed is "vái trabalho" which translates as "go and work." The conviction here— and the instruction — is for each individual to take responsibility for his or her own healing: and that involves work, not miracles. These were the main things that I got from being there, together with the opportunity to work in an extremely focused environment which is blessed by a feeling of optimism and faith; a belief in the possibility of healing, even in very extreme circumstances. Quite the opposite to many hospitals, which I often found to be places filled with fatalism and despair.

The Casa provided a place where I could go and spend hours and days and weeks: I was fortunate to be able to go five times during the year after my diagnosis and I spent a total of about eighteen weeks there. There was no "miracle" healing for me; I was told on my first visit that I would be healed, but could never get an answer to my questions about how, when or where this might be achieved. (Did it mean returning to London for conventional surgery? I was never told either "yes" or "no.")

Not everyone experiences things at the Casa in the same way. Some people visit only once for just a few days. A tiny minority do experience an apparently 'spontaneous healing.' Others stay for months and months and show no apparent physical improvement—although it is impossible to assess what im–provement they may be making on spiritual levels.

A lot of serious work was done while I was staying in Brazil. During my first six-week trip I made a key decision: not to hide behind the cancer, or to use it as an excuse for denying responsibility for my feelings or actions. I was encouraged in this by Carl Simonton's book which includes a very telling exercise that asks you to list the possible "benefits" of having cancer. My list included: avoiding work I found difficult; getting myself looked after; and escaping punishment for my wrongdoings. Simonton encourages you — as a matter of survival — to find ways of addressing these issues that do not depend on having (or keeping) the cancer.

Q: Apart from going to the Casa de Dom Inácio, what other spiritual work did you do?

CHRISTOPHER: The other area that I explored was Tibetan Buddhism. I was able to take advantage of the contact I'd already made with the work of the Tibetan Lama Sogyal Rinpoche (who is best known for his book *The Tibetan Book of Living and Dying*.) I spent time among Buddhists who believe that death is not necessarily a bad thing; it is something we don't need to be afraid of and can actually prepare to do well. Tibetans view illnesses such as cancer, not necessarily as life-threatening, but as a "wake-up call," bringing our attention to problems of spiritual neglect. There's also a belief, similar to that at the Casa, that it's possible for us to access a divine source of healing energy. In the case of Tibetan Buddhism, there are specific practices to help encourage and achieve

73

this: specific meditation practices, visualisations and mantras.

The Tibetan Buddhist community at Dzogchen Beara in south-west Ireland encouraged and guided me in how to use a meditation practice called "Vajrasattva," which simply employs the idea that a source of divine light, of healing energy, can be brought into our bodies and can help cleanse us and heal us. (There is a lot in common between some Buddhist meditations and the sort of "visualisation" techniques advocated by many healers and doctors, including Carl Simonton. You certainly don't have to be a Buddhist to use these effectively.)

While I was in Brazil the first time I spent many hours listening to tapes of Sogyal Rinpoche teaching about Vajrasattva: apart from instructing me in how to do the meditation, these deepened my understanding of the importance of feeling regret, owning up to my mistakes, then apologising and asking for forgiveness. I did this meditation every day, sometimes for hours, but certainly every morning and night during the time when I was most ill. And I continue to do it now.

The other idea that came from Tibetan Buddhism that I found helpful was the notion of "karma." For me the concept of karma had a lot to do with accepting the interconnectedness of things within my life and seeing that, put very crudely, I could have accumulated the negative effect of my own negative acts, be they in thought, word or deed, by commission or omission. This helped me to focus, at a philosophical and spiritual level, on the fact that some of the causes of my illness lay within my own life; in my way of living and in my actions.

Q: What do you mean exactly?

CHRISTOPHER: I was forced to see the areas in which some of my actions had been hurtful to those close to me. I began to realise that, powerful as I might have become in the world, I was often failing to act with a proper sense of awareness and responsibility. A failure that sometimes led to unwitting abuse of those around me.

Buddhism is very strict in encouraging us not to hurt other sentient beings, and tells us that in the act of hurting others we accumulate negativity within and for ourselves. The idea that in hurting someone else you hurt yourself, was a very important part of understanding how I'd come to wound myself so much.

What Buddhist thinking and teaching did for me was to provide a springboard into an area of emotional work, of counselling and therapy which became – together with spiritual healing at the Casa and Buddhist meditation – the third key corner at the base of a sort of healing pyramid, seeming to reach heavenwards, in which the spiritual and emotional underpinnings of my illness were tackled.

The goal of the emotional work was to help me release some of this distress so that I could think and act as clearly as possible in the midst of my predicament; and to help me reach again and again for a firm belief in my right to live. This was the emotional counterpart to the spiritual cleansing; the two went hand in hand, and for me this involved facing up to some very difficult and uncomfortable realities about myself.

I do realise that, for many people who suddenly find themselves very ill, the idea that there is going to be an emotional dimension to physical illness may be one of the hardest things to contemplate, to be open to, and to agree to do something about.

Q: Why?

CHRISTOPHER: Because it could very easily feel like you're blaming yourself for getting ill. Most religious practices have built into them the idea of redemption or forgiveness; so there's an immediate benefit to owning up, to repenting. But facing your worst thoughts, your failures, your demons in an emotional, therapeutic setting, where there are is no ready-made offer of any redemption — beyond that which you are able to fashion for yourself — means that it can be very tough.

I was lucky to have willing friends who were prepared to dive in alongside the more trained and already skilled counsellors, including Sally, who took the key initiative of organising the support group. So I was blessed with a great opportunity in which to do this very challenging emotional work. I can see that most people do not have that ready opportunity. But nonetheless, I would urge three things upon anyone facing a serious illness:

One is to try psychotherapy in some form, to acknowledge the need to express the difficult emotions that come with illness. To do that needs both space and committed attention, ideally from a professional.

Second is to organize a support group of some kind among your friends and family. The people who are most intimately connected with you and your illness should have the opportunity to share among themselves their hopes and fears, as well as some

"...the idea that there is going to be an emotional dimension to physical illness may be one of the hardest things to contemplate, to be open to, and to agree to do something about."

of the practical information about the business of helping you to get well again. A support group, even if it doesn't function as a psychotherapeutic or counselling support group, can provide solidarity for those most intimately involved, helping them not to feel alone in the face of the illness.

The third thing is to acknowledge the needs of the principal care givers: those who are involved most fully with you and your illness, to encourage them to take the time and space to release their own fear and confusion, to replenish their hope and strength, and to get them to be as clear as possible about how they can help you without damaging themselves.

Q: Did the spiritual work and emotional therapies make a difference to your physical well-being from the outset?

CHRISTOPHER: When I was first diagnosed I had no clear-cut ongoing physical symptoms. The symptoms crept up on me in the months that followed. As the tumour grew, and started to impinge upon other tissue and nerves, so the pain grew. Five or six months after the diagnosis, I was in almost unremitting pain of a highly disabling order. I could hardly sit or stand, and I certainly couldn't sleep. Sometimes I could bare-

ly speak because all my attention was being sucked into a black hole of pain. I got very sick. I was doing all these things to help my healing but I was still getting sick.

Q: This didn't make you lose faith in what you were doing?

CHRISTOPHER: No. Other people have been comforted by the fact that, for me, things got worse before they got better. The split between the medical and alternative points of view was a difficult one to deal with, given that I was in terrible pain and the people close to me did not always share my conviction that the healing was possible without surgery. At this stage there was apparently objective evidence in the form of the X-ray and scan results, that in spite of everything I was doing, the tumour appeared to be getting bigger. On the night of the scan results there was an emergency meeting of the support group that lasted into the early hours of the morning. It was then that I took the decision to open myself completely to what conventional medicine had to offer — including surgery. This change of heart was an important point of surrender for me, turning around a very old pattern of rigidity. Up until then I had been quite dogmatic in my view that I was going to do things my way, and my way wasn't going to include submitting to surgery.

By this time the tumour was of such a size and in such a position that it wasn't operable without completely devastating and mutilating surgery. The recommended medical plan was to use radiotherapy and chemotherapy in an attempt to shrink the tumour and to make it surgically operable. So, paradoxically, the consequence of deciding to accept surgery was to grant me more time without surgery. I decided against the chemotherapy (because I wanted to avoid something that seemed to me likely to deplete my whole system, including my immune system) but accepted the proposed course of radiotherapy. That provided a focus and a time-frame during which all my other healing endeavours could be intensified.

Q: How did this work?

CHRISTOPHER: I was prescribed a seven-week course of daily radiotherapy, followed by a wait-and-see period of up to a further eight weeks to see the effect of the radiotherapy on the tumour, prior to any surgery. I decided to bracket the course of radiotherapy by making two more trips to Brazil, a two-week trip immediately prior to the radiotherapy, and a three-week trip immediately after it. I continued alternative treatments, adding hypnotherapy, osteopathy and hyperthermia, a form of treatment that is hardly accepted at all by the medical establishment in Britain. It's a centuries-old concept of healing lesions or tumours with heat. I rented one of the a hyperthermia machines, and Sally and a private nurse took the responsibility of administering the treatment every day through the whole seven weeks of radiotherapy.

Q: What happened next?

CHRISTOPHER: By the end of the course of radiotherapy, the pain was starting to diminish. I had been on very heavy-duty painkillers, including morphine, which at the worst time weren't touching the pain, it had gotten that bad. (At this point my only source of relief was marijuana.) But now the pain started to go away, and I took the last painkiller on the plane to Brazil, at the end of the radiotherapy. After three weeks in Brazil the pain had entirely gone and when the MRI scan was done back in London it showed that the tumour had completely disappeared. This was on 26 May 2000, nearly seven months after the diagnosis.

"...I do know, without any doubt, that conventional medicine alone could never have healed me."

This was seen by all the doctors as an exceptional outcome for conventional radiotherapy: it is almost unheard of that a tumour should go completely. It's not clear who, or what, should take the credit for this. The doctors take the view, as they must, that the radiotherapy was responsible and I was very lucky to get such a spectacular result. I don't know for sure that my body needed the radiotherapy (it is still recovering from the unwanted side-effects,) but my mind certainly needed the act of surrender involved in accepting it. And everything else undoubtedly played its part. But I do know, without any doubt, that conventional medicine alone could never have healed me.

Subsequently, the advice that I got from a number of the alternative practitioners was that the work had to carry on in order to complete the cleansing process, to allow my body to recover from this enormous battle that it had fought, and to continue boosting my immune system so that it could return to total health.

It was not until six months after the disappearance of the tumour (and two more visits to the Casa de Dom Inácio) that "João de Deus" told me I was healed, saying to me 'It is finished. You can go now.' It was exactly a year and a day from my first arrival at the Casa. By then I had developed the firm conviction that health, and staying healthy, must become a way of life. And what I feel I've now made is a life-long commitment to taking care of myself and my body.

Throughout my journey from sickness to health, I was blessed with incredible love and support. Whenever I asked for help it came. Above all, I had my beloved Sally. Somehow,— God only knows how — she found the courage and the strength to set aside her own pain and grief and fear to be with me night and day, whenever I needed, as a source of loving attention and intelligence. In celebration of survival, the strength of the human spirit and the healing power of love, we got married on 7 July 2001, fourteen years from the week we met.

MAURO DOS SANTOS SILVA

PEDRO LEOPOLDO, MINAS GERAIS, BRAZIL
YEAR OF BIRTH: 1961
Grade School Teacher

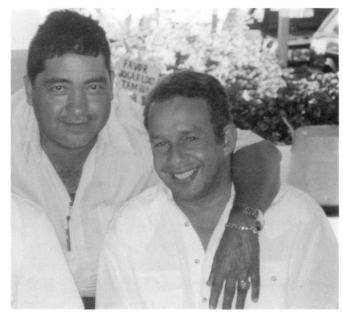

Sebastian and Mauro

Mauro was skin and bones when he first came to the Casa in March of 1993. His mother, who accompanied him, thought that her 33 year old son was being eaten up by cancer. So did the rest of the extended family. Mauro's doctor had told him he was in the final stages of AIDS. Mauro had been given a blood transfusion years ago which was infected with the HIV virus. Seeing John of God was Mauro's last hope.

For hours he stood in line, like everyone else, waiting to consult the Entity. The Entity was brief. He prescribed herbs and said what everyone hopes to hear, "I will cure you." Even though Mauro believed in the power of the Entity, he couldn't believe what he had heard. As soon as he was ushered out of the Entity's room, he doubled back and returned to the assembly hall to stand in line again. Hundreds of people passed in front of the Entity before Mauro saw him for the second time that day. This time, the Entity was right to the point, "Didn't you hear what I said? I said, *I will cure you.*"

Mauro left the Entity's room and went to the men's room, adjacent to the assembly hall. He was spent. He lost all muscular control, collapsed to the floor, soiled himself, and was almost unconscious when a visitor discovered him.

Sebastian, João's secretary, was alerted that there was a man dying in the men's room. Sebastian immediately went to Mauro. Deeply shocked by the sight of this man, so close to death, lying in excrement, Sebastian prayed to Mother Mary for assistance while he put Mauro in the shower. With labored breaths, Mauro tried to warn Sebastian, "Stay away. I have AIDS." But, Sebastian continued washing him up, finally wrapping him in a clean sheet, carrying him into the surgery room, and placing him on a gurney.

"With labored breaths, Mauro tried to warn Sebastian, 'Stay away. I have AIDS.'"

Sebastian told me,

I wanted to at least let him die clean and in a sacred place, not the floor of a bathroom. I also offered him a meal. I wanted him to die with some sense of comfort. At first, Mauro declined all food, but after I continued to encourage him, he had two bowls of the blessed soup. Then, he asked for rice and beans and eggs—the typical food from his state of Minas Gerais. I had the kitchen staff prepare this special meal for him. After he ate this, he had water and two deserts. Then, he got off the gurney, stood up and walked into the Entity's room, where he filled a water bottle with blessed water energetically charged by the entities. Soon after, Mauro left with his mother to go home, a twelve hour drive.

I didn't see how this man could live. I had seen his body. It was covered with open sores. There was hardly anything left of him. He had almost completely wasted away.

Forty-five days went by. I was sitting at my desk one morning and I felt a presence behind me. Then, a pressure on my face and neck. I looked in back of me and saw Mauro's face. I thought, 'O my God, the man's ghost has come back to haunt me. What should I do to get him away from me?' I was very scared. My heart was pounding and my hair stood on end. But, Mauro grabbed my shoulders in an embrace, laughed and reassured me, 'I am alive! I am here with my mother and father. Come outside and meet them. I am not dead!' I went outside and we all hugged and laughed together.

I was so happy to see Mauro alive. I feel like I am Mauro's spiritual father. Even though I had spent very little time with him, I felt strongly that I wanted him to live.

When I met Mauro it was September 21, 2001. He had been using the Casa herbs and staying on the Casa diet for eight years. He had also been returning to the Casa every forty five days, to see the Entity, sit in current, and bring others to the Casa for healing. When Sebastian called me into his office to meet Mauro, I met a strong, handsome, well-dressed, and very present man. It was easy to believe that Mauro was a successful professional. Sebastian gleamed with pride as Mauro answered my questions about what had helped him heal:

I tried one AZT pill, years ago, but it was too expensive for me to continue on it. I never used any conventional medication for AIDS after that one pill. I just saw the Entity, sat in current, and took the herbs. I also didn't drink anything dark—like Coca cola or coffee. I never had surgery or used any other treatment at the Casa. For the last seven years I have had no flu, no sickness or any symptoms at all. My physician at home recently said there is no trace of AIDS in my system. I am no longer HIV positive.

I asked Mauro what has been central in his healing. He said,

I focus on being alive, being here in the present moment, thinking positively. I continue to work teaching math, science and biology to kids from seven to fourteen years old. I look after my mom and dad who are old and need my help. I share the power of my healing process with others, and encourage them to do their healing journey. I lead a normal life, including sexual relations.

Along with the discipline it takes to follow my treatment, my faith has been essential. I am a practicing Catholic. I believe in God. I also believe that the energy of God is accessible to us through Jesus Christ who transmits his love through beneficent entities who help us to heal. So, like 80% of Brazilians, I go to a Spirit House for healing. Here I feel more personally touched by the love of God through entities like Dom Inácio and Dr. Auguste.

Toward the end of our interview, Sebastian looked at Mauro with great excitement in his eyes. He said, "The Entity wants me to tell you some-thing very special. He checked you today and sees no evidence of illness in your spiritual body, or any part of you." Mauro lit up with joy. It had been eight years of ongoing work.

As I turned to leave Sebastian's office, Sebastian said to me, "Now, in your book you don't have to mention what sexual preference Mauro has." I looked back at Sebastian, wondering if he had judgment about gay people which I had missed. Mauro looked a bit uncomfortable for the first time. I was new to the Portuguese language and was relying on a translator. Suddenly, the situation felt very awkward.

Clarifying himself with a twinkle in his eye, Sebastian continued, "If people look at Mauro's photo and realize that he is available, there might be a lot of people who come down here looking for him! You might want people to know that Mauro is heterosexual."

Sebastian's playing with us was actually a bridge to a broader invitation:

We want people to come. The Casa is open to anyone, regardless of sexual preference. We don't care if people are gay or straight or what they do with their sexuality. That is their business. We attend to spiritual healing. All are welcome here.

DONNA MOSEMAN
LEBANON, NEW HAMPSHIRE
YEAR OF BIRTH: 1951
Artist, mother, wife

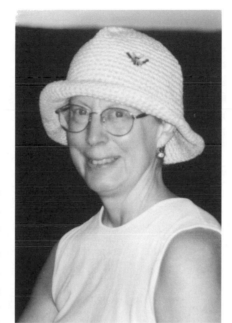

June 27, 2001. Donna was sitting on the porch of her 1886 Victorian house when I drove up. Her hair was now evenly half an inch high like a new mown blonde lawn, arching over her softly feminine face. A red string, signifying her Buddhist commitments, was tied around her neck, discretely tucked into her T-shirt. To get out of the sticky heat we went into the cool of her living room, through the door she had hand-painted with the Buddha of Compassion hovering over a calm ocean. We had an hour to talk before Donna's ten year old daughter, Hester, brought a friend home for some watermelon.

Donna's energy is still low. She can't walk far before her breathing becomes labored. In 1995 her doctor noticed calcifications in a duct in her breast but there was no palpable lump until 1998. At that time Donna began working more closely with an oncologist and elected to have a lumpectomy. In the winter of 2001, the cancer metastasized into her lungs.

Donna's first doctor had not recognized the severity of Donna's condition. The doctor was monitoring her through a sequence of blood tests and allowing Donna to approach the pre-cancerous condition with natural herbs. In hindsight, Donna believes a stronger protocol, such as chemotherapy or radiation, would have been more appropriate. She began a more conventional protocol, using Herceptin, a drug which goes directly after the cancer cells, in the Fall of 2000. Since Herceptin has been so effective, Donna now follows her oncologist's advice, using a variety of drugs and chemotherapy to treat the cancer in her breast and lymph nodes, and, more recently, in her lungs.

When we first met in Abadiania, April 17, 2001, Donna was approaching the cancer from a spiritual perspective as well as continuing conventional medical treatment. Despite not feeling strong, she had been inspired to go to Brazil to visit the Casa for two weeks with her friend, Susan. Ten weeks later, she was quite philosophical:

The cancer has been a spiritual journey. It has taken me into the depths, and also brought me to appreciate the simple beauty of my life in a way I never had prior to having cancer.

I was not miraculously cured in Brazil. In fact, in early May, right after I returned from Brazil, I was so weak I could barely feed myself. My chest was so congested I had to be on oxygen 24 hours a day for three weeks. Everything was turned inward. It was just me and the disease. I know some people at the Casa say, 'It can get a lot worse before it gets better,' and that 'healing is a journey.' I held on to that point of view during the worst of it. Then, my oncologist put me on more aggressive chemotherapy. It's helping me a lot. I am feeling really optimistic now.

I can't say for sure what is happening but I have been steadily improving since June 9th. That was the day I lay in bed beside my still sleeping husband, Jim, and prayed to God that I become healed.

Seconds after, a miracle happened. I could feel my chest clear, my breathing suddenly become open and free. My husband woke and said, 'Your breathing hasn't been this open for months.' I quickly got out of bed to walk around, wondering if the healing was total and I had my full energy back. Well, I was better, but not completely. That's okay, I really do know it is a pro-

cess of getting better and better each day. But, the openness in my chest was truly amazing. It seemed to happen so quickly, right after my prayer.

I had never really prayed before *directly* to God. I have meditated. I have been on spiritual retreats doing concentrated mindfulness training. But prayer has not been part of my life. When I was in Abadiania something opened up in me. I felt a direct connection to God and spiritual forces. I can now bring that feeling of connection into my prayers.

I remember my second day in Abadiania, right after the invisible surgery, I felt bubbly and happy, truly joyful as I was walked home to the inn. The surgery itself was not memorable. João de Deus said prayers and then left, I guess. I just remember feeling very tired, almost like I couldn't move, during the session. Then, right afterwards, when I went out of the surgery room, I was loving to look at the light, the flowers and trees. I was enjoying moving my body, feeling a sense of freedom and lightness. A butterfly flew toward me. I felt deeply loved and deeply connected. I began to think of my future and how I wanted it to be.

The gift I received at the Casa was the knowingness that there is this other realm of spirits and we are cared for. It is not just me caring about God, it's God loving me, directly and personally.

"I had the courage and took the time to enter into the truth of my life."

I asked Donna to tell me more about her healing. I was interested in knowing how her life was changing:

Since Memorial day, I have been painting again. I have combined the triangle symbol and the beautiful rainbows I saw at the Casa with things which are part of my life in New Hampshire—the morning doves I watch from my porch, a red cardinal, butterflies, different flowers which are brought to me each week by my neighbors or Hester's music teacher.

I used to be very active, constantly going to art shows, taking my daughter places, going to the Mindfulness Center to meditate, being involved in my community in various ways. I thought being limited to sitting down on my porch for lengths of time would be hard. Actually, I used to meditate on the porch for relatively short periods of time; now, I sit, sometimes for hours, simply appreciating life. Different birds fly by. The flowers and trees change shape and color. The weather is constantly changing.

After Donna shared about her healing and the deepened peace which had entered her life, I asked her to tell me more about her experience in Abadiania. Handing me a beautifully decorated, archive quality scrapbook, she continued:

The photographs I took when I was in Abadiania are very telling. I participated fully in all the activities. There were hundreds of people at the Casa when I was there; but, not one of my photographs shows a person. I have sunsets, buildings, streets, trees, the bench where I sat in the garden of the Casa, the door of my bedroom at Hotel Amazonas, and sculpture I saw in Brasilia. But, no people.

It seems I was just perceiving the skeleton of life, the bare bones. I felt very alone in Brazil. My husband and daughter were at home in New Hampshire. I missed them. I painted by myself in the Casa gardens in the afternoons. Susan and I had separate rooms, and she was caught up in her own health issues. I was feeling a litle less than 50% of my normal energy level. I don't speak Portuguese. All these things added to my loneliness.

Then, I realized that I hadn't really ever told myself that I had a life threatening illness. Imagine that! Six years of being sick with cancer, and I hadn't thought about dying. While I was at the Casa it started to become more real, I had the courage and took the time to enter into the truth of my life. I didn't have additional symptoms or complications, but the bare bones of my situation were—I have cancer that has metastasized and I might die.

In the current room, sitting in meditation, surrounded by other mediums and visitors who were also meditating, I finally went directly into the center of my situation. I engaged the illness, really let myself feel that I was very sick. I went even more deeply into the spiritual nature of the illness, going directly into my own truth, past all the ways I had been distracting myself. You know, my mother had died of breast cancer when she was 75 years old, in 1984. She had her first bout with the cancer in the 1960's. That was a time when physicians did radical mastectomies as a matter of course. My mother had suffered terribly. I had to confront my memories and feelings around her dying.

One of the most helpful people I met in Abadiania was "little João," one of the translators. He came over for a meal at our inn, right after I had surgery, and talked about how healing has to be taken on by the person who is ill. It's not just João de Deus doing the work. The sick person has to grapple with the philosophy of Spiritism, meditate often, look inside, eat the right foods, confront the illness and the roots of the illness, etc. It is work. After that lunch I realized that I had been wanting to heal for my daughter's sake, so she would have a Mom. During my respite after the Entity's surgery, I decided I wanted to heal for *me*, because *I* want to live as well as be here for my daughter and husband.

Knowing that Donna had been a dedicated member of the Mindfulness Community of Thich Nhat Hanh, a Vietnamese Buddhist monk, I was interested to know what she thought of João de Deus and the community of people who visit the Casa:

I didn't feel especially close to João-in-Entity. He wasn't very available. Consultations lasted seconds. I don't fault him for it. He had hundreds of people to care for. But, I didn't have time with him and he didn't say very much. I certainly never thought it was all up to him to make me well. I also don't have a sense of urgency about him or the Casa, like I just have to get back there because it is him that will heal me.

As Donna spoke, I was aware of the gentleness with which she deals with herself. She was not forcing her speech, but rather taking time, allowing her story to emerge. Not far away from her words was a bit of raspiness, the slightest touch of an obstruction in her breathing.

She appreciates all the different parts of her healing process:

Along with the conventional drugs I've used to confront the cancer, two elements, the connection to God I had at the Casa, and my home community, have been the most significant.

My own community in New Hampshire is very strong. I have a great oncologist: She is very supportive; gives me information; tells me about possibilities; and then, respectfully, asks me *what I want to do*. The neighbors bring me and my family food and flowers. My child's school community organized to bring us dinners every night. When my husband worked and I was really sick and needed someone here 9 am-4 pm every day, someone in our community came over, helped me do what I needed to do and kept up with the housework. I've also received very good healing work from a variety of body workers in Vermont and New Hampshire.

I don't know if I could have made the progress I have made without having been to the Casa. I was truly inspired there, especially in the current room, and I still feel that the entities are working with me now, in New Hampshire. I am not alone. I have help. I am being loved. *I have faith* that I am on the road to the recovery of my health.

As of December 23, 2001: Donna continues to have her ups and downs. Her pace is slower than it used to be before she had cancer. From time to time she is weak and needs extra oxygen. She can not be as independent and she has to rely more on her family. However, she is again driving her car, active as a mother, artist, wife, and community member.

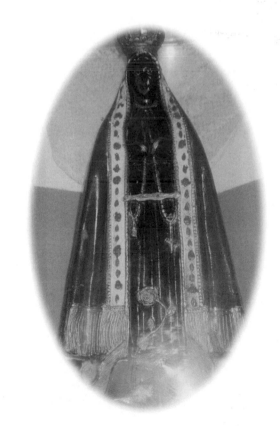

NARADA MUNI DAS

(BIRTHNAME) LENNY RADER
ALACHUA, FLORIDA
YEAR OF BIRTH: 1948
LENNYRADER@CS.COM
Distributor of herbal remedies from South America

Wearing white t-shirts and muted orange dhotis (loose pants typical of India) a white dot painted on the center of their foreheads, one hand enclosed in a prayer bead bag, Narada and his friend, Tribhuvannatha, stood out in the crowd of people at the Casa de Dom Inácio. I'm sure I wasn't the only person wondering how these people from the Hari Krishna movement had found their way to João's sanctuary in Brazil in early March, 2001.

On my first day at the Casa, I had seen Tribhuvannatha fall to the ground, unconscious, as he stood watching the orientation in the morning, one in a crowd of over three hundred people. As the Casa volunteers gently carried him to the recovery room, I noticed how very thin he was. Narada recalled that Tribhuvannatha had been ill with stomach cancer at that time. As Tribhuvannatha was looking at the photo of Dom Inácio in the assembly room, he had become overwhelmed with the presence of entities and fallen to the floor in a profound state of bliss.

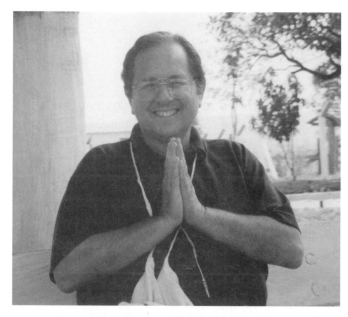

The entities often work with people who are standing in the assembly room, or meditating anywhere on the Casa grounds. I was warned to not be surprised if someone fell down during the assembly. Jabuvanath has the ability to feel the entities working on him in a very dramatic way. Other people say they feel nothing, but sometimes discover the thin line of a scar on their bodies, evidence that they had surgery without consciously being aware of it.

Narada was diagnosed five years ago with Hepatitis C, a virus which is blood borne. He contracted the disease in 1971 from a blood transfusion he received during surgery for removal of a cancerous tumor. Western medicine knows of no cure for Hepatitis C. Treatment involves rest. Drugs, like Interferon, which

"I had been given a mantra the day before in a dream, and I was repeating it to myself. 'Love protects. Love nourishes. Love heals. Love forgives. Love is grateful. Love is Divine.'"

are hard on the liver, are usually prescribed. (Combination therapy with Ribavirin is now used which often has severe side effects...including major depression and aenemia.) Narada believes the chemotherapy actually challenges the body still more than the Hepatitis. Patients must curtail or limit sexual activities, as the virus can be transferred to others through saliva or blood. Patients usually die from progressive degeneration of the liver, cirrhosis. The severity of Hepatitis C is monitored through blood tests which track the elevation in enzyme levels and viral counts.

Narada has not taken any conventional drugs for his hepatitis. In July, 2001, he began to take herbs from the Amazon Rain forest. However, he assigns his progress in overcoming hepatitis to the work that he has done at the Casa de Dom Inácio.

On his first visit, in March, 2001, the Entity told Narada that he needed surgery that day. Narada was then faced with the decision about whether to do visible or non-visible surgery:

I wanted to experience the physical surgery. For me, it was an act of faith. So, I volunteered for visible surgery.

The process began when I was sitting in the surgery room waiting for the Entity. I began having visions for about half an hour which were very intense. I saw Jesus Christ amidst throngs of people. Radha and Krishna, the Divine couple who represent the female and male aspects of God, were there. So was the founder of the Hare Krishna movement, Srila Prabhupada.

Then, I was ushered into the Entity's room. I was already in an altered state, quite unaware of time and space and very relaxed. The Entity took my head in his hands, and, before I knew it, he had a six inch long surgical tool up my nose and was twisting it. I felt no pain at all, but I was aware that the procedure was happening. I have done spiritual practices which help me disassociate from my body for thirty-five years, so being quite detached from body sensations is not new for me.

Immediately after that procedure was over I was led to the assembly room. I had been given a mantra the day before in a dream, and I was repeating it to myself. 'Love protects. Love nourishes. Love heals. Love forgives. Love is grateful. Love is Divine.' As a result, I had very little fear.

I was standing against a wall in front of the assembly when the Entity used a surgical knife to make an incision in my lower abdomen. I had very little discomfort. I do remember the cut as a jolt to my nerv-

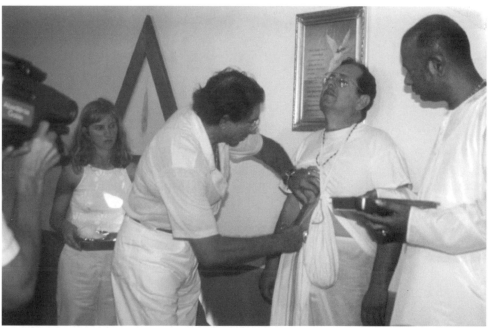

João de Deus operating on Narada at the Casa

After this surgery I felt enraptured in bliss for days. I rested and meditated in my room, then returned to participate in the current after 24 hours. The most important part of my healing process since that surgery has been sitting in current, meditating and praying on my own, and continuing taking the herbs prescribed by the Entity.

ous system, but my attention soon turned again to dramatic visions. I saw myself lying prone in front of God in the form of Radha and Krishna. Real tears of gratitude were streaming down my face.

The incision the Entity made was about three inches long and just below my liver. I bled only a few drops. The Entity put his fingers in my body through the incision and moved his fingers around. I believe he was changing the energetic patterning in that area of my body. He did not take anything out of my body. After a minute or two, he removed his fingers, briefly wiped around the incision with a cloth, then, sewed it up with a few stitches.

I have continued to receive unexpected gifts which have amplified the healing. For example, I was intensely curious about how João incorporates an Entity. I wanted to see it. One morning, I was standing in the assembly room during the orientation. João came out of the current room, said a few words in Portuguese (which I don't understand) and then pointed at me. I came up to him. He took hold of one of my hands with both of his hands. I closed my eyes. In a few seconds, João, the man, left his body and another Entity came into his body. I could feel the shift in the energy during the incorporation (as if he had been told that I wanted to experience it.) It is hard to describe what I felt during those seconds.

Yes, there was a distinct energy. I felt transported to a causeless, non-judgmental love for all living things. He dropped my hand after less than a minute, and turned to the other people he was going to operate on. *I stayed in this non-judgmental state of mind for a number of hours. I am sure it is this energy that helps transmute sickness.*

In August, when I had my annual blood test, my enzyme level was in the normal range for the first time in five years, and the viral count had decreased 75%. I still have a way to go, as clinically I am not healed, but the results thus far border on a complete remission of symptoms. I also measure this through major differences in my energy level. I am able to do most things now, like take walks and do normal chores, where I was severely limited just a few months ago.

The second time I came to the Casa, it was in mid-summer, 2001. I brought some people with me and helped them in their healing. I was told I would be completely cured. I was also told that I am being prepared to do healing work with the entities. This is very exciting for me, and something I want to do.

This time (September, 2001) I have seen the Entity once. He told me that my work is in the current room, and by giving to others I will be cured.

Narada and I met again in the Casa garden to speak about the terrorist attack on New York City and the Pentagon. I was struck by Narada's ease and joy in referring to his religious beliefs, and, at the same time, his willingness to converse and be open to my perspectives. Still, his certain alignment with his own perception infused everything he said. And, he did not hesitate to share this certainty with me—especially as it regards healing:

We have tremendous power in our minds which affects the body. Everything starts in seed form on a subtle [spiritual] platform. Every disease. Every joy. Everything. What one learns here at the Casa de Dom Inácio is that the spiritual and physical are deeply intertwined. We can effect physical change by doing spiritual work. We can study how spiritual work effects physical health here. We can integrate the physical with the spiritual, that is, truly become spiritual beings, with spiritual intentions, using the body as a vessel to do our work.

SHARON LECKIE
NEW ZEALAND
YEAR OF BIRTH: 1960
Wife and mother of two

DREW UMBER
YEAR OF BIRTH: 1952
NEW ZEALAND
Administrator/Counselor: helping teens realize and manifest what they most want to do with their lives, including attending the college, or vocational training of their choice.

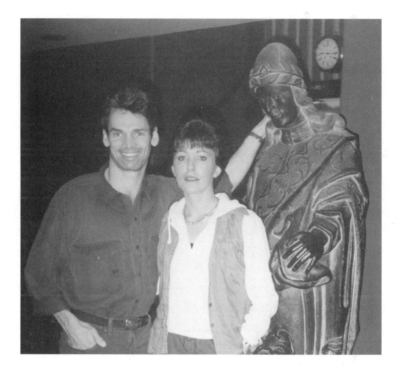

In 1995, Sharon, age 35, had been diagnosed with arthritis and degeneration of the hip, spine and neck joints—the result of her hip bones being too big for their joint sockets at birth. Among other things, she had tried massage, laser treatment, acupuncture, physiotherapy, Reiki, and herbal supplements. Nothing had turned the tide of the degeneration and increasing pain. Almost all exercise was now impossible. She felt hopeless and depressed. Happily married, with two children under ten, there were few fun activities she could share with her family. Her physicians said hip replacement surgery was the only thing conventional medicine could offer her.

Sharon's friend, Drew, at 38, had chronic Lymphocytic Leukemia. This type of leukemia is rare at his age and there is no cure available from orthodox medicine. Drew's doctors held out little hope.

In an e-mail, Sharon described how she decided to go to Abadiania and also included excerpts from her journal:

I had 100% faith in this trip to Brazil, even though I knew very little of what I was getting myself into. My mother, who had recently died, came to me in my meditation, and stressed that this trip must take place in August, 2000. I decided to use the money she left me to pay for my own trip and Drew's expenses, too, since he was limited in his ability to work. We defied all other logic to go.

TUESDAY, August 8, 2000

When we checked in at the airport in Auckland, Drew was limping badly, and was in a lot of pain from a growth which covered the complete groin area and half way down his thigh. This lump appeared two weeks before the trip, and even though the specialist wanted to administer aggressive chemotherapy, Drew had declined. Drew's skin color was between yellow and gray.

I had a huge knot in my stomach. What on earth was I doing? The odds of Drew surviving the flight were very poor. As Drew had so few red blood cells to provide oxygen, he would most likely have immediate cardiac arrest when the plane gained altitude and the cabin was decompressed, reducing the oxygen level. Drew asked my brother and me to witness and sign his will, so he could give it to his Dad at the airport. It was an emotional leave-taking with many tears.

There was nothing to do but put our faith in the spiritual help around us. As the plane climbed Drew and I held hands tightly and prayed that we would have the support we needed. When we reached 5,000 feet and Drew was breathing great, we knew we were going to be okay. Seven hours into the trip Drew said 'I am so happy, I can't sleep.' My relief was immense.

We negotiated the long flight, the overnight in Rio, airport transfers and taxi to Abadiania with few problems, and arrived at our inn.

WEDNESDAY

The people we have met here are wonderful, there is a great feeling of peace and love at the Casa. You feel warmth to your heart and soul the moment you arrive.

After waiting in line for two hours at the Casa, we finally filed through to be received by the Entity. When my eyes met the Entity's for a brief moment, I felt him look beneath the exterior straight to my soul, an incredible feeling, amazing and terrifying all at the same time. I could not stop crying.

After a rest, we returned to the sanctuary at 2 pm to sit in the first current room to meditate. I found it very hard to meditate for long periods, as I am not used to this.

Each evening I went into a deep immediate sleep, dreaming of the past and issues I had not confronted and dealt with. I would spontaneously wake from my sleep about 2 am, and would sit for two hours dealing with these issues and tossing them away. Only then would my sleep resume.

> God helps those who help themselves, but not those who limit their action to asking for help.
> — from Kardec's "The Spirits' Book"

THURSDAY

Drew had an 'invisible surgery' this afternoon. Upon entering the current room, Drew's emotions overflowed, and his tears poured out. He then experienced short heavy breathing and was told by Patricia, a translator, that his discomfort was quite normal, and that the operation had already started. Just after he sat down, he felt as if a five inch cut was made inside his thigh. It was subtle and deep. This strange phenomena lasted only a couple of seconds. Assistants then helped him up, and led him to lie on a bed to receive the rest of the operation. For nearly a minute his actual heart felt like it was being kneaded forcefully from every angle, as if to squeeze out negative feelings and hurts. He cried silent tears for the next ten minutes and then it was over.

Drew was then led to the recovery room to be watched over by the volunteer they call 'the Angel,' who attends to any wounds, covers you in blankets, speaks and sings softly in the most beautiful voice, all in Portuguese. The pain in his groin and thigh had changed from a gross throbbing pain to only a thin sharp pain where he had felt the cutting. Later that day, Drew was able to walk without a limp for the first time in four weeks. The swelling of the leg was also reduced immediately.

FRIDAY

I had my first invisible operation. After sitting quietly a few moments, suddenly I felt like two fists were going into each of my hips, first the left and then the right, working and prodding and trying to realign my hips, then the pubic bone. Tears streamed, and I felt very overwhelmed by the presence of God. I felt I was still in the process of the surgery when I was told the surgery was complete.

I went to stand but could not, feeling light headed, nauseous, and heavy. I must have been coming out of the spiritual anesthesia. I also had severe groin pain. I was instructed to take five deep breaths, breathing in the positive and light, and breathing out the negative and lower feelings. Still very shaky, I was taken to the recovery room to rest.

The soothing voice of 'the Angel' volunteer made me feel I was truly in the presence of an angel. While I was in the room, many people were brought in. All fourteen beds were full, as the Entity had been doing many visible surgeries. One lady had gauze over both eyes where they had been scraped. The gauze was bloody. When she left 45 minutes later her eyes were fine and only slightly red.

*"Warmth and love spread throughout my whole body with
an unusual peace and serenity."*

After having some vegetable soup, I was driven back by taxi to my inn. I had been told not to carry my backpack or exert myself after surgery. I spent the afternoon in bed. It is hard to explain, but I felt weak, tired, disoriented and in pain, alternately with a feeling of being engulfed by spirit. Warmth and love spread throughout my whole body with an unusual peace and serenity. It was a truly wonderful experience.

That night I was delirious, feverish and ill. I later discovered a scar from the surgery that ran from my groin to my hip, about four inches long. I was instructed to bathe it with the blessed water from the Casa. This scar was to fade five days later, as the swelling and the bruising left.

SATURDAY - TUESDAY

On Saturday I awoke with a sore and swollen groin area. Throughout the four days I had varying amounts of pain which had almost disappeared by Wednesday.

Drew and I spent time meditating in the garden. The feeling in the Casa grounds is totally amazing— serenity, peace, upliftment and beauty. I think I could stay in this place and time forever.

I continue to receive emotional healing from dealing with my dreams every night. I sense this is required to heal physically. I did some spiritual reading and writing.

WEDNESDAY

I went back before João-in-Entity later in the morning for a review. He took my hand and said "Come back at 2 pm," to be reviewed by a different Entity. I was both scared and exhilarated. Drew was also told to return that afternoon. Maybe we have to see the Entity that first worked on us? I don't know.

I had amazing feelings when I went for my first crystal bed treatment. I felt my bones being stretched four ways; my feet being pulled and stretched; the base of my spine, my third eye and eardrums had intense pressure and I felt burning in my stomach. Again, even though it was sometimes painful, I had an incredible peaceful feeling.

Drew is very well; everyone has noticed the return of normal color to his skin. He wakes early (which is unlike him) feeling very energized. He has not needed his daily rests. He feels weary after the Casa each day, but after a shower he feels fine. He has stopped all night sweats. His mind is now working clearly, and very rarely does he get short of breath. Amazingly, the white flour, cheese and sugar that has been in many of the foods has not bothered him. The mass in his leg has reduced to a small hard center, red and inflamed, about the size of an egg which still hurts when he walks. The rest of the leg is fine. Right bladder pain is now all clear. Drew is loving the meditation time. He said he experienced balance, warmth, and centeredness for 45 minutes in a crystal bed treatment he had today.

THURSDAY

I went into the operation room for another scheduled surgery this morning. Nothing much happened at first, and then a blinding pain in the back on my left side at the base of the spine, like a red hot poker, went straight through to my left ovary, very intense. When we were told to leave the room, like the first time, I felt nauseous, light headed, and my head ached. I was given a prescription for three more bottles of herbs. Back at the inn in the next hour, I felt intense pain, bordering on unbearable, which eased after two hours.

Drew had another operation this morning which was very subtle. He felt empowered and uplifted. His physical pain has been replaced by a quiet, centered internal space. He was told that this centeredness would be his strength, and that he can participate more actively in his own healing now. He was also told that the lump would disappear as he lay his own hands on the area; also, by his participating in his healing, he was learning lessons which he would use to help others in the future. His lump has reduced by one fourth and was less painful.

By 5 pm, my body was very relaxed. I felt a lot of movement in my joints, like they are going back into the right place.

FRIDAY

I awoke with no pain, something has definitely changed. I feel different, lighter, like anything and everything is possible. Although there is still a weakness and tiredness, I am clearly healing.

This morning the Entity spoke to the crowd telling them that some of them had not taken their herbs. He asked them to return to their homes, take the herbs and then come back, as the herbs were for spiritual treatment before surgery. It was amazing to see that these people thought the entities wouldn't know, and that they could hide not following instructions.

I went before the Entity and told him that my hips were still sore and that I could not return to Brazil another time. He touched my hip and said 'You will be fine. Sit in my current room and I will drain the pain from your hips.' I also asked, 'What spiritual path should I take to help others?' Once again the Entity responded, 'Sit in current. Our spiritual paths cannot be revealed to us by someone else; we must find the answers.'

The Entity told Drew to come back in November and to sit in the Entity's current room to meditate today.

"Our spiritual paths cannot be revealed to us by someone else;
we must find the answers."

Drew knows that the level of emotional and spiritual work he does before this next journey will impact the level of healing he receives.

We both had very powerful meditations. After five minutes of meditation I experienced a surging pain lasting two minutes from my back down through my hips, literally draining downwards. After that I had no more hip pain.

João-in-Entity operated visibly on many people in the line passing before him. It was an incredible sight to see. The Entity cut across the back of one man with a scalpel and started squeezing around a large purple cancerous-looking lump. He squeezed the flesh, and after a short time he used some scissors and extracted four lumps, which looked like tumors, after which the man collapsed into a chair and went to the recovery room. There were other operations where tumors were removed that would fill a jar.

We had a small party for our inn-keeper, Martin, with a band and a cake. Drew organized singing 'Happy Birthday' in all the languages of the guests at the inn.

SATURDAY

We left Abadiania today with lots of hugs and photos with our new friends.

TUESDAY

It is wonderful to be home and be back with my family, but part of me will always be connected to Brazil. Drew has returned a different man, his skin is normal color, as are his eyes. Even after all the walking, the lump has reduced another quarter with less inflammation. He has high energy levels and is walking well, no longer fragile.

Drew said, 'The whole trip has totally blown me away. It was far more profound and effective than I could possibly have expected. I feel unbelievably softened and warmed on the inside and spiritually enlightened. I am still moved to tears with gratitude.'

Not everyone suffers with the degree of pain Drew and I experienced in Brazil; many people have no pain. As I was unable to return to Brazil in the near future, I received much of my healing in a short, intense period of time. Drew also needed to get rapid healing, as his disease was so far advanced. You receive what you ask for, although not everyone can be healed in one visit.

TWO WEEKS LATER

Judging by the expectations of modern medicine, Drew was expected to die on our trip. The doctors in New Zealand have been amazed that he no longer has the large lump on his leg. They are unable to explain it.

AFTER SIXTEEN WEEKS, DECEMBER, 2000

Drew has returned from his second trip to the Casa able to work again. Before he went he was dangerously unwell. He said, 'The Entity instructed me to have whatever the doctors were offering me to take away the symptoms while I carried on with the meditation work.'

Since my return I have had two surgeries from the entities followed with twenty-four hours of some pain, a temperature and leg swelling. Now, the swelling is gone. I have far more flexibility with my hips, much less pain and a much healthier attitude to life and spirit. My children have commented that I have come back a different person— they like the changes. The experience has not only changed my life but inspired me to help others. I am 80% better and now lead a totally normal life.

DECEMBER, 2001

Drew writes: 'On and off since December, 2000, I had chemo and blood transfusions and Prednisone, and then followed up with some lighter chemo back here in New Zealand. I have refused to take stronger chemo, (intravenous Fludarabine). Instead, I'm trusting the process. Life is really rather wonderful.

I have just returned from my fourth trip to the Casa. All of my symptoms except a little breathlessness from the low hemoglobin count have practically disappeared and I'm living a completely normal life again now with work, romance, hour-long walks each day up and down the beach—I look and feel normal.'

FERNANDO JOSE CORREIA VICENTE
PORTUGAL
YEAR OF BIRTH: 1962
EMAIL: FERNANDOVICENTE@CLIX.PT
Computer aided designer for engineers and architects

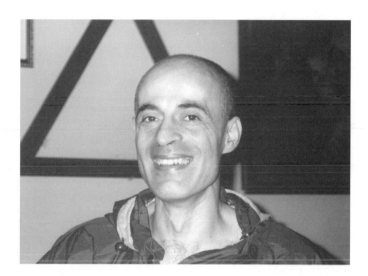

Fernando hesitated at the dining room doorway clearly charting his path through the sea of tables. It was hard for him to walk a straight line, and harder still to hold a cup of tea or manage eating a bowl of soup. When he sits down his arms and hands shake uncontrollably. Two steps, and then a lurching forward into a run, is his normal gait. The dining room was too short to accommodate his stride. He had to slow himself, grabbing onto the backs of chairs for stability, as he made his way to the buffet table with his wooden bowl.

Susan, an Australian woman staying at the inn, helped Fernando to salad, chicken and rice, and put his full bowl at his place at the table. Because he was especially nervous today, Fernando ate without utensils, leaning his head directly into the bowl for his food. Fluids were tipped into his mouth for him, or he managed with straws, leaning toward the cup on the table. "Looks like the advanced stages of Parkinson's disease," I thought to myself. Curious that only his arms and legs tremble, while his head and trunk seem stable and centered.

The next day, I sat down beside him in the morning sun before going into the current room to meditate. I said,

"Hi. I noticed you just arrived at the inn where I am staying. I'm here writing a book. I'm interested in Brazilian Spiritism." I paused, hoping he would tell me why he had come to the Casa.

Fernando surprised me. He said, "I am here to let go of my ego. I don't like the way I am with other people. I judge too much. I want to love more fully."

He was direct, non-blaming, elegantly simple. He didn't say a word about his physical condition, as if it was incidental. He felt his real suffering stemmed from what he considered an impairment in his ability to accept himself and others.

"We are all here to learn to love. How we appear, and the state of health we have is inconsequential. Deepening in our capacity to love is all that matters."

All spirits have been created equal by God; but some of them have lived more, and others less, and have consequently acquired more or less development in their past existences. The difference between them lies in their various degrees of experience, and in the training of their will, which constitutes their freedom, and in virtue of which some improve themselves more rapidly; hence the diversity of aptitudes that you see around you.

—from Kardec's "The Spirits' Book"

Immediately, I knew Fernando was a teacher for me and many others. His non-verbal message was extremely clear: We are all here to learn to love. How we appear, and the state of health we have is inconsequential. Deepening in our capacity to love is all that matters.

A few days later, my last day in Abadiania, Fernando allowed me to interview him. I figured this would give me permission to ask for his physician's diagnosis (as if Fernando's reason for being at a healing center was too spiritual to be *real*). We sat in the small reception area of our pousada in overstuffed chairs stiffly covered with naugahyde. He began with his childhood:

My father was a perfectionist. He never admitted failure. Because of my father, I learned to have a very determined will. Even as a child, I used to tremble. I think it was in response to the stress of being around my dad's expectations.

By the time I was twenty-four, I had overcome the trembling, but, one day, I felt a chill along my whole spine. Since then I became more nervous, always trembling a bit, especially when I was being observed. When I was thirty I was working hard cleaning swimming pools. I used to clean twenty pools before 2 pm, never stopping for a rest, or any food. Suddenly, my body went rigid, my muscles hard. I was almost completely paralyzed.

I waited, thinking my condition would go away by itself. I trembled intensely for fifteen days before I went to see a doctor. After a month of tests at the hospital, I was diagnosed with 'essential tremor,' an ideopathic condition—meaning the origin is unknown and the treatment unclear. Allopathic physicians offered drugs, but I declined. Instead I turned to homeopathy, acupuncture and spiritual work to help me understand and treat the core of the problem.

Acupuncture has given me some relief. When I was thirty-three years old I saw Anton Jayasurea, a world-famous acupuncturist in Sri Lanka. He had no diagnosis for me, but I felt that the one hundred treatments I had with him were helpful. A Dutch acupuncturist gave my condition the name of 'Wind on the Liver.'

When I asked Fernando what he did for himself to treat his condition, he said, "I cry a lot. It helps release some of the tension." Clearly, his running everywhere also released tension, kept his muscles toned and his body oxygenated. Fernando also studies the Course in Miracles, the channeled teachings of Jesus. He said:

I am trying to trust a higher power than my ego. I think my tremor is the result of a strenuous effort I make to control myself and my life. I want to stop resisting life and instead release, surrender to be one with all that is. You can't do that if you reject yourself, or fight being yourself. Any resistance creates more obstacles. If a drowning man surrenders to the water he can float and save himself. If he resists drowning, and fights for control, using his energy to flail around, he exhausts himself and drowns. I am learning how to surrender.

Suddenly, Fernando's voice dropped and tears filled his eyes. I felt as if I was in a psychic elevator with him as we descended from the eighth floor to the basement, in a split second.

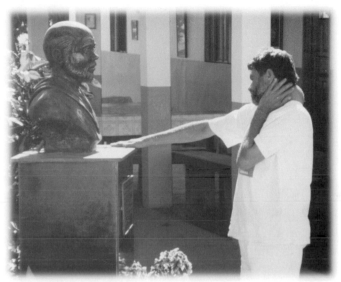
Man praying by sculpture in garden of Casa

My life is barren if I don't love and don't connect. My heart needs warmth. I need to learn to connect with others without any calculating, or strategizing, to get *what I think I need*. I need to be willing to let some beneficent power outside myself work on me. I am at the Casa de Dom Inácio to learn more about this kind of surrender.

Brazil has an important role to play in world spirituality. Brazilians value a pure connection to the Divine. When you visit here, you can see this purity, learn to bring it out in yourself, and receive the light of God more readily. I want to be healed by this love.

Tears now erupting from his eyes, Fernando said,

"If I do not become more of an instrument of God and his purity, my life is a loss."

Fernando's sincerity and intense desire to surrender more deeply into love moved many people.

Within two days of his arrival, two generous men gifted him with room and board for his two months in Abadiania. Fernando had made the two day trip to Abadiania by himself, with just enough money to cover a two month stay at our inn. (Imagine, he must allowed strangers to help feed him along the way.)

> *"The fatality which seems to shape our material destinies is, then, a result of our free will?* You yourself, have chosen your trial; the severer it is, and the better you bear it, the higher you do raise yourself....The aim of trial is to leave to màn the entire responsibility of his conduct, since he is free to do or not to do [good or evil]."
> —from Kardec's "The Spirits' Book"

When Fernando heard that the paraplegic man sitting next to him one morning, eating soup, was a venture capitalist (investing in business for profit), he turned to him with a mischievous smile, "You should invest in me." To which the man replied with affection and humor, "Seems like a shakey investment." Laughter spilled out of everyone at the table.

At some point, looking at a table of ten people, each with his or her different grave illness, you drop every idea of what *should be*, appreciate the drama we call life, and laugh with tears of joy and love streaming down your face. A few minutes later, you hold a cup for your neighbor, knowing that without your help, he can not drink.

I have included Fernando's story because in many ways it is the unending story of every soul who is using this life to grow into being a more loving being. Fernando and I passed each other only briefly —he was arriving in Abadiania just as I was leaving. Yet, Fernando seemed to articulate so beautifully the real essence of why people suffer, and what they need to do to end their suffering. Disease, conditions of the body which make us "abnormal," anxiety, depression —all of these may be incidental, just a bit of baggage to manage, in our larger quest for love. No healer, no spiritual sanctuary, no culture can cure us of our inability to surrender more deeply to love. However, each person we meet, whether he or she is a healer, or a person looking for health, can be an important part of our journey. It is up to each one of us to allow these spiritual alliances into our lives.

Ten weeks after I met Fernando he wrote to me from Portugal,

> It is obvious that I suffer, but I wouldn't exchange the birth of my true identity for some kind of bodily relief. I am aware that what is good and attractive for my ego is not necessarily so for the growth and emergence of my true self. Deep down I think I have a great trust in the justice of life. ✿

PART FIVE: LIFE AT THE CASA DE DOM INÁCIO DE LOYOLA

Early in the morning, an arresting visual tide of humankind's physical and mental ailments moves slowly toward the Casa —individuals of every age, body type, and skin color. Almost everyone is confronting AIDS, cancer, heart disease, paralysis, mental retardation, fear, addiction, or some other kind of illness. When people first meet they ask, "Where are you from?" Next, "Why did you come all this way...what are you here to heal?" We talk about the physical problems we want to address, but our eyes reveal our longing for spiritual wholeness, our hope for a deeper connection.

Like other visiting health professionals, I thought I was drawn to visit the Casa because I wanted to witness João-in-Entity; to volunteer my own energy in the work; and to increase my ability to help others. I had no idea how much I would be moved by the people I met, the courage and the capacity to surrender to spirit which I saw dramatized all around me, night and day.

Connection with the Holy Spirit

As an agent of extraordinary healing who transcends normal limitations, João-in-Entity is called "The Miracle Man." He is also an ordinary man who works all day, and doesn't go home until the Entity who incorporates within him has consulted with the last person waiting to be seen.

To focus on João solely as a spectacle, a miracle man, is to miss an essential part of what he offers. The work of the Casa is not to make João more special in the eyes of the world, but to remind everyone of us of our ability to connect with spiritual realms. Remember, not in Entity, João repeats everyday , "It is God, not me, who does the healing." João's greatest gift is to reveal our close connection to evolved spirits and *the energy we call God*. His work calls us to drop our limiting beliefs about our separation from spirit; to let go of our fears and reach for our closeness with God. João and his volunteers encourage visitors by often saying, "In God, all things are possible."

João's work is *spiritual healing*. It goes to the root cause of the problem in the spiritual body and eliminates it there. This psychic surgery may not deal with anything we would call physical; instead, it eliminates the intent, or seed, which caused the physical problem. Recall the phrase in the Bible: "In the Beginning was the Word, and the word was God." In this case, in the beginning is a subtle intention which is not physical, and the intention manifests later as a physical reality. In *Faith healing* the healer enters into the patient's body energetically and removes the problem on the manifest level. Spiritual healing and faith healing are thus subtly and profoundly different.

The reason João, both as himself and as the Entity, always invites visiting doctors to be near him as he does visible surgeries is to assist them in realizing their own potential in spiritual healing; to learn how to bring spiritual healing into their own work in clinics and hospitals; to become vehicles of the spirit and pass that ability on to others. João's welcoming film-makers and photographers to record his work is, similarly, aimed at disseminating the power of spiritual healing.

Many Christian traditions teach that it is only Jesus and the apostles who had extraordinary gifts of healing. For the last two thousand years religious leaders have considered those who claimed to have extraordinary healing abilities to be blasphemers, heretics or charlatans. I am not suggesting we liken John of God to a Christ or one of the apostles, but instead, that we consider that ordinary people, like João, can choose to have the Holy Spirit flow through them. It is not only our potential; it may be our next step in evolution. João may be guiding us in the transition to our next level, that of being in direct communion with the Holy Spirit, which not only helps us become more whole, but empowers us to be healing forces in the lives of others.

Using the term Holy Spirit should not have to limit us to only consider one part of the Christian trinity. The qualities associated with the "*Holy Spirit*" are embodied in the sacred language of many spiritual traditions. They are never ascribed to a human being as the energy of the Holy Spirit is too vast to be contained in one individual or one name. Buddhists use the word, Dharma, to refer to *the living spirit of truth*. Hindus conceptualize the spirit which animates creation in Shiva and Shakti, a god and goddess. Ancient Indian texts, the Vedas, conceptualize infinite wisdom as *pure awareness*. Muslims conceptualize the spirit of God as Allah. Thus, human beings of all cultures create linguistic constructs to give shape to the sacred power which is beyond being contained.

Spiritist doctrine ascribes the qualities of the Holy Spirit (pure compassion, infinite wisdom, creative energy, and a desire to be of service to others) to *perfection*. When we stop identifying with our personalities, and we identify with our highest potential, allowing the Holy Spirit to move through us,

"...the manifestation of the Spirit is given to every man."

we embody this perfection. In Part Three you 'read how the Entity has initiated physicians—bringing them into a more expanded energy field where they can focus and intensify energies for healing.

Olga Worrall, a gifted healer from the USA who was often called on to help physicians, feels that people who are given the gift of healing have a responsibility to share that gift. In her book, *The Gift of Healing: a Personal Story of Spiritual Therapy* (1965), she refers to the Bible to illustrate that Christianity accepts healing as well as diverse expressions of spirituality:

> *Now, there are diversities of gifts, but the same Spirit.*
> *And there are differences of administrations,*
> *but the same Lord.*
> *And there are diversities of operations,*
> *but it is the same God which worketh all in all.*
> *But the manifestation of the Spirit is given*
> *to every man to profit withal.*
> *For to one is given by the Spirit the word of*
> *wisdom; to another the word of knowledge*
> *by the same Spirit;*
> *To another faith by the same Spirit; to another*
> *the gifts of healing by the same Spirit;*
> *To another the working of miracles; to another*
> *prophecy; to another discerning of spirits;*

> *to another divers kinds of tongues; to another*
> *the interpretation of tongues;*
> *But all these worketh that one and the self same*
> *Spirit, dividing to every man severally as he will.*

> *—I Corinthians chapter 12, verses 4-11*
> *King James Version, The Holy Bible*

I invite you to consider John of God as a guide in our personal evolution, Spiritism as a language to conceptualize this evolution, and the community around the Casa as individuals reaching for union with the Holy Spirit. A young Portuguese man, familiarly called "little João" so as to distinguish him from João de Deus, came to the Casa in May, 2000, a heroin addict in despair. It took him many days to stop using drugs, and almost a year to heal his wasted body with the help of the entities. It was the loving nature and the kindness in the human and spiritual communities, which inspired him to change his life. The next stage in his healing is to help others without asking for or accepting remuneration. Selflessly, he makes himself available as a translator for English speaking people who come to the Casa to consult with João-in-Entity. Little João's goal is to become a medium, and after a year of dedicated service and study, he has become a knowledgeable

104

and kind guide to travelers visiting Abadiania for the first time. Volunteers at the Casa, like little João, serve the healing of others, with sincere loving compassion. This service is an expression of their own journey of purification and spiritual growth.

> *In what way can Spiritism contribute to progress?* By destroying materialism, which is one of the sores of society, and thus making men understand where their true interest lies. The future life being no longer veiled by doubt, men will understand more clearly that they can insure the happiness of their future by their action in the present life. By destroying the prejudices of sects, castes, and colors, it teaches men the large solidarity that will, one day, unite them as brothers.
>
> —from Kardec's "The Spirits' Book"

The Natural Environment

The hours I spent exploring the natural world around the Casa both on foot and horseback, were always a pleasure. The central plane, where Abadiania is located, is over three thousand feet above sea level. The air is clean. The stars seem very close. The sunrises and sunsets are dramatic light shows— as are the thunder and lightening storms which periodically crack the skies, often leaving rainbows in their wake. In March the hillsides were lush with tall green grasses. The fragrance of Eucalyptus trees scented the air on sunny days. Up to one hundred green parrots flew together, like fast-moving clouds, darting around the sky at sunrise and sunset, chattering and squawking. Roosters crowed at dawn.

The hill on which the Casa sits is believed to be formed mainly of quartz crystal. Like smaller crystals, it both stores electro-magnetic energy and facilitates communication. Perhaps the crystal is a keeper of the spiritual intentions of the entities, the volunteers, and all people coming for healing, who believe they can be helped by the entities of the Casa.

The streams that flow out of and around this same hill of crystal are believed to be a special source of healing. The Entity sometimes prescribes sitting under one particular waterfall as part of treatment. One must have permission from the Entity to visit this waterfall, as well as be accompanied by a Casa volunteer while there. This insures that the place will continue to be treated with respect.

The unusual geological nature of Abadiania, and the caring stewardship of the place, may also be one of the reasons the Casa is considered a "portal," facilitating our connection to the spirits who do healing work.

A Place of Learning, Service and Community

The Casa may nurture visitors in ways that we can not measure or be conscious of. Little João believes that there are invisible spiritual realms around the Casa where our spirits study and expand their understanding of ultimate truth. He implied that this learning happens when we are in altered states of consciousness, such as meditation or sleep. Little João studies Kardec's writings on Spiritism in weekly classes with other Casa staff and volunteers. In this way he tries to make the learning, happening on a subconscious level, more a part of his conceptual understanding. He encourages visitors to continue to study their own spiritual books as part of their healing work.

All the Casa staff encourage visitors to study spiritual books, but do not proselytize. Whether we are spiritists or not, the study of spiritual books helps us structure our thinking, so that we can align both our thoughts and our actions toward spiritual evolution. João, the man, smokes cigarettes but, in Entity, he implores people to stop smoking. João, too, is in a process of aligning his thoughts and his actions with his spiritual wisdom. At this point, the best way he can do it, is to dissociate from his body and serve others as an unconscious medium. As he continues to evolve, perhaps he will learn to align himself more completely so he can remain conscious, deliberately choose to be an instrument of God, and continue his healing work while he is fully present. One morning, in April, 2001, João confessed to those of us in meditation at the Casa that he realizes he is in a process of growing to become an even greater agent for spiritual healing. He said, "It may take me many more lifetimes to be as good as Chico Xavier."

During this confession, I became poignantly aware of the power in the spiritual community of the Casa. No one can grow spiritually or perform great works in a vacuum. The spiritual community of the Casa, with thirty-two paid staff and over two hundred volunteers, called the daughters and sons of the Casa, support the Entity's healing work. This is readily apparent when you first come in to meet the Entity and you see twenty Casa volunteers meditating in the ante room, called the first current room, alongside visitors; and then twenty or thirty volunteers meditating in the Entity's consultation room, called the second current room. These experienced meditators are creating energy through their immersion in the Holy Spirit in order to support the Entity in his healing work, and the transformation of each visitor in his or her healing process.

It is said that manifesting our highest potential is as difficult as balancing while walking on the sharp edge of a sword blade. We need others, attuned to the path, to help us stay in balance. Spiritual allies are a boon and deserve to be treasured because they help us along our way. The community of the Casa de Dom Inácio, including João de Deus, is a place to be treasured both as a healing center and a university, serving all who want to grow spiritually.

Following is more detailed information which will help you picture what it is like to visit Abadiania, and how the Casa de Dom Inácio functions.

On Wednesday, Thursday, and Friday of each week, João de Deus comes to the Casa to see people in the morning after 8 am and in the afternoon starting at 2 pm. There is a break for lunch from 12-2 pm. It is requested that people who come to consult with the Entity wear white clothing, suitable for meditation and respectful of the spiritual nature of the place, i.e., skirts or slacks are preferable to short shorts and halter tops for women.

Orientation Talk

The first event of the morning is an orientation given by someone closely associated with the Casa. The talk begins soon after 8 am. The assembled audience is first greeted formally, often by Sebastian, João's secretary and right hand man, who welcomes everyone with both warmth and a sense of serious intent, respectful of the difficulties many have had traveling to Abadiania. Sebastian has worked closely beside João for more than fifteen years and carries a lot of authority in the management of the Casa. Another of João's assistants then speaks about the work that is done at the Casa. On some mornings, depending on the makeup of the assembly, the orientation talk, first spoken in Portuguese, is translated into English.

During the orientation people are strongly encouraged to follow any instructions given by the Entity. Cooperation, over time, with the treatment offered, is an essential part of healing. Everyone is asked to keep their arms and legs uncrossed while at the Casa. This allows energy to pass through the body unobstructed, which helps the group, as well as João, have access to a greater quantity of healing energy. Silence during the sessions is requested. There are dietary restrictions which apply to people who are prescribed herbs as well as those who have surgery. These dietary restrictions need to be maintained for the duration of the time people take the herbs, at least forty days. People who have surgery are requested to leave the Casa after their operation and not return for 24 hours. They are open and vulnerable, and it is strongly suggested that they rest quietly for at least a day. Those who have either visible or invisible surgery are requested to abstain from any sexual activity, including masturbation, for forty days. This is to reserve life energies for healing. Those who have surgery are also requested to return for a review, giving the Entity a chance to prescribe the next level of treatment.

Everyone is invited to have free vegetable soup, served at the dining area at approximately 11 am on Wednesday, Thursday and Friday— after the morning session is over. Made with a base of winter squash, this soup is hearty and easy to digest. It is also blessed by the entities, and helps with healing.

Following this invitation and the instructions, there are often testimonials given by a variety of people from diverse cultures, who have dramatic stories of their own healing through the entities' work. Even if you don't follow the language spoken, you can feel the strength of conviction in the people, as well as their spiritual devotion. Often, the one who tells a story, also leads the group in the Lord's Prayer, followed by a prayer to Mother Mary.

People of all religious traditions are welcomed. Even though there are Christian prayers and Christian iconography on the walls, there is great respect paid to those of all faiths. João has said, "The only thing we do here is open our faith in God." Reflective of the diversity of our world, the orientation talk can range from loud, evangelical passion, to quiet, tender communion. It depends on the person who is assigned the talk on any specific day.

Watching Visible Surgeries

Sometimes visible surgeries, performed by João-in-Entity are done in the assembly hall after the orientation. Surgical tools, like Kelly clamps (scissors with tips that are bent at a forty degree angle) and sterilized knives, are used as well as paring knives common to any kitchen, and an ordinary sewing needle and thread for suturing incisions. Invisible surgeries, in which no visibly invasive surgical procedure is performed, can happen any time, day or night, during your stay in Abadiania, or even, after your stay. João says that the work is really done on the energy body of the individual, and visible surgery is for those who would not allow themselves to heal unless they had visible surgery.

When João first walks out to the assembly before operating he has not yet incorporated an Entity. As João Teixera da Faria he may talk to the assembly about mundane matters for a few minutes, or speak about the work of the Casa.

After his talk, he incorporates an Entity. This process may be barely perceptible. Often João holds the hands of an assistant for a moment with his eyes closed, and then, on opening his eyes, relates to the group in a more detached way. Sometimes the incorporation is very dramatic. I have seen him stand in the center of the platform where he does his surgery, with his hands by his sides facing forward, ready to receive. Then, his body is taken over by some spasms, his fingers gripping his palms, his breathing full, his eyes and face wincing. After a few minutes he looks noticeably expanded, as if he has taken on more weight and more light, simultaneously.

Casa staff and volunteers who have attended João for years say that identifiable characteristics of the Entity he embodies show up immediately. For example, the volunteers sometimes tell visitors who ask them, "It is Dr. Auguste here today." Visitors to the Casa can plainly see the character changes, even if they can't recognize the specific Entity being incorporated. The Entity's demeanor ranges from that of a rigid perfectionist, to someone who is exquisitely compassionate and gentle. After incorporation "he" looks at the audience briefly and then goes to work.

Generally, the Entity attends people one by one who have lined up for visible surgery first. After incorporating the Entity and performing visible surgery, he may also walk through the assembly room, followed by a couple of assistants carrying surgical instruments on metal trays, and spontaneously work with other individuals. *He does not force surgical interventions on anyone who refuses the work.*

Physicians who are visiting are invited to stand close to João while he operates, and then report what they see to the assembly immediately after the procedure is finished.

When a surgery is complete, the person who has been operated on sits down in a chair. Two strong volunteers then lift the person in the chair and take him/her to the recovery room to rest on a bed. Wounds made in surgery are cleaned and dressed in the recovery room by the volunteers who work there.

The Recovery Room

The recovery room is a private room lined with 14 beds in a quiet corner of the sanctuary adjacent to the assembly hall. The room is only used to attend to people who have had visible or invisible surgery, and need a quiet place to rest and be attended to, prior to leaving the Casa.

There are several staff members who stay in this room, watching over the people who need care,

Map and layout of the Casa

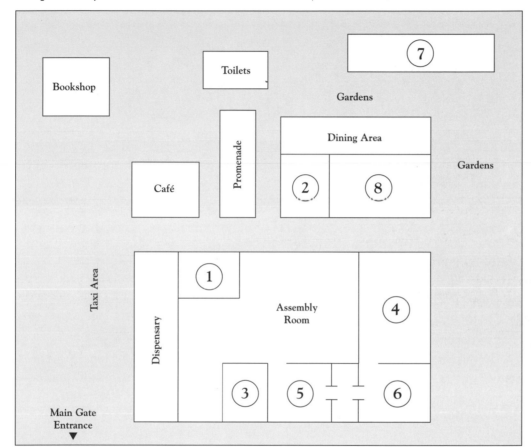

Key:
1) Storage of crutches, wheelchairs & protheses which were discarded after healings
2) Secretary's Office
3) Recovery Room/Infirmary
4) Surgery Room
5) First Current Room
6) Second Current Room
7) Treatment Rooms: Crystal Beds
8) Offices & Kitchen

attending to wounds if need be, providing water and food and/or emotional support, as necessary. It is not unusual for additional prayers to be said in the recovery room.

The Surgery Room

After the visible surgeries are performed, João-in-Entity leaves the assembly hall and goes to do the invisible surgeries in the surgery room. This room, with a door to the outside, is adjacent to the room where João-in-Entity consults with individuals. The surgery room is lined with benches in the center and beds around the perimeter, to accommodate those who can not sit. Attending this room are a few of João's assistants.

After having invisible surgery in this room, patients are guided outside to the secretary's office. Photographs are taken of each person; names, addresses, and contact information is collected. The photographs are placed in the Entity's prayer basket. In this way his work continues on each person after they leave the surgery room.

The Current Rooms

After the Entity does visible surgery and invisible surgery, the rest of the people in the assembly form lines to enter into the room where João-in-Entity does his consultations. There is a line for people coming for the first time. Another line for people who have already consulted with him once. Another line for those needing a "review" after previous surgery, where the Entity pays special attention to the progress that has been made since the surgery, and considers the next step in treatment.

When the Entity is finished with the invisible surgeries, he goes into his consultation room to meet visitors. The lines proceed in an orderly fashion through the "current rooms," where there are typically between fifty to one hundred people meditating and praying. There are no instructions given on how to meditate or pray. People are encouraged to follow their own ways. However, it is suggested that for some of the time you sit with your hands on your legs, palms upward, in an open position. This is a re-

ceptive position, in harmony with keeping yourself open to inspiration and help from spiritual sources.

What is the general character of prayer? Prayer is an act of adoration. To pray to God is to think of Him, to draw nearer to Him, to put one's self in communication with Him. He who prays may propose to himself three things: to praise, to ask, and to thank....[you] are always free to invoke the assistance of God and of good spirits to help [you] to surmount your [problems]."

"Is there any use in praying for others?" The spirit of him who prays exercises an influence through his desire to do good. By prayer, he attracts to himself good spirits who take part with him in the good he desires to do.

—from Kardec's "The Spirits' Book"

A sculpture of Mother Mary is in each current room as well as a few other religious or inspirational pictures on the walls. A large clear quartz crystal sits in a prominent place on a table near João's chair in the second current room. As you walk through these rooms it is not unusual to palpably feel the energy and positive intent of the meditators. Typically one volunteer for the Casa is saying prayers out loud to

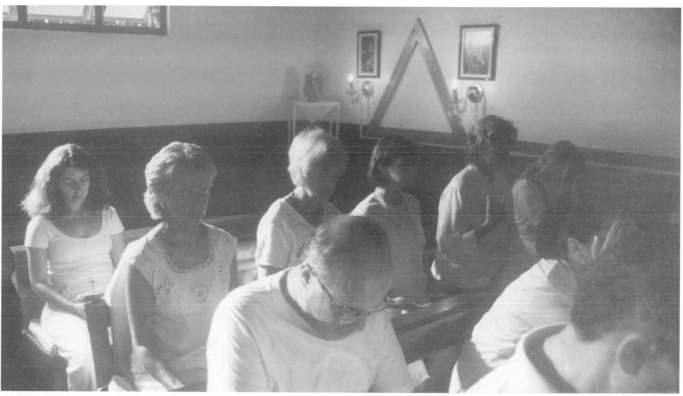

Meditation in the Second Current Room

help people stay focused. Music is played through speakers in each room. The music varies from classical to inspirational to popular Brazilian. This variety of music is selected to assist people to stay present in the here-and-now.

After the first current room one enters the "Entity's room," also called the "second current room." João-in-Entity sits in a chair against a wall facing the entry. Translators attend him as needed. A number of Casa volunteers sit facing the Entity, eyes closed, meditating. These people, recognized as mediums by the Entity, have been asked to dedicate their work

to assisting him with the people he works on. Some visitors are also invited to meditate in this same room after seeing the Entity for consultation. There are rows of benches provided, all of which face into the center of the room.

When you are meditating in the current rooms you are requested to keep your eyes closed. In fact, you are told that the entities can not help you in your work unless your eyes are closed. When the sessions are over in the morning and afternoon, you are offered a small glass of water to drink which has been blessed by the Entity. Then, it is time to leave.

Consulting with the Entity

It is suggested that you continuously meditate on the problem you are experiencing as you wait in line to see the Entity. When your turn comes, the Entity will first look at you, without having heard your question. As he looks at you, he sees your condition on all levels: physical, spiritual and emotional. This is referred to as "seeing your blueprint." Sharon, who tells her story in Part Four, explains, "The entities can read everything—your thoughts, past lives, karma, intentions and current activities. When you come before the entities, you literally open your soul."

João, the man, was asked, "Do the entities know everything about us?" He responded, "If they work with the energy of God, then they know everything." The Entity is then in a position to prescribe herbs or treatments as well as answer your questions. Questions can revolve around any issue which is important to you. After giving you your prescription, which may include surgery, you are typically invited to sit in the first or second current room to meditate. The consultation generally lasts a matter of seconds. More time is taken when surgery is performed, but the procedures are usually brief.

The Entity deals with each person in a very individual way, according to the problem, the intention of the visitor, and what he feels called to do. João, the man, recently said, "Everyone who passes in front of the Entity will receive exactly what they need. If your spiritual treatment is not finished when you leave the Casa, distance will not separate you and the work will continue, wherever you are."

People who have little intention to follow the Entity's advice are sometimes dismissed quite quickly. For example, an Australian woman and her daughter had a very negative attitude toward the whole Casa. They were concerned they would be given herbs, and would be asked to discontinue their habit of drinking alcohol. The Entity first looked hard at them, prescribed nine bottles of herbs (a supply lasting three months), and then waved his arm, indicating they go to the current room—without any further explanation. By sitting in meditation, surrounded by the positive energy of other mediums, they would hopefully confront themselves and understand that they needed to participate actively in their healing.

Two or more translators are available to facilitate English, Spanish and German speaking peoples interaction with the Entity. It is advisable to make contact with the translator prior to seeing the Entity, in order to clarify your question. This is often done before formal sessions begin in the morning and afternoon. The translator will write your question on a piece of paper, then give it back to you. When you approach the Entity, after waiting your turn in line, the translator will be present, will ask for the paper with your question, will translate your question to the Entity in your presence, and then write his answer for you on the back of the paper and return it to you. In this way you have a record of what is said, and can ask for further clarification from the translator after the session, if you need it.

About Payment for Services

The Casa is dependent on donations for maintenance, but does not ask any fee for the Entity's services. There are no charges for the translators, sitting in the current rooms or using the recovery room. *They want the work of the Casa to be available to everyone, regardless of one's financial resources.* However, there are several clearly marked boxes set up around the Casa to receive donations.

João, not in Entity, is an ordinary man, who makes his money as a rancher, miner, and owner of a car dealership. He is Catholic, currently not married, and lives in a town thirty minutes drive from the Casa. With a handful of devoted staff and vol-

unteers, he also manages the business of the Casa: making sure there are supplies for the herb room and the kitchen, and maintaining the sanctuary and its garden areas.

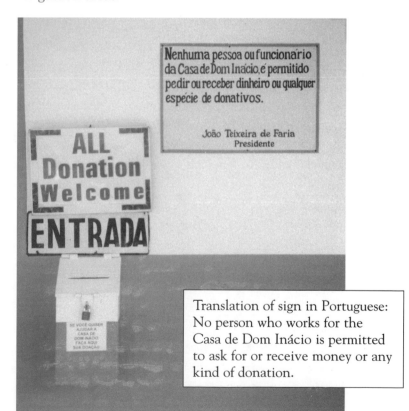

Donation Box

Nenhuma pessoa ou funcionário da Casa de Dom Inácio, é permitido pedir ou receber dinheiro ou qualquer espécie de donativos.

João Teixeira de Faria
Presidente

Translation of sign in Portuguese: No person who works for the Casa de Dom Inácio is permitted to ask for or receive money or any kind of donation.

A Magic Bullet or Miracle-Grow?

There are some people who come to the Casa searching for a "magic bullet." They want a surgery, a healing, an herb, or something that will make all their symptoms and their problems disappear forever. Right now! They decide to come to the Casa for a day or two—enough time to see the Entity, get the magic bullet, try the food, and leave. "If he's the real thing," they think, "then he should be able to do what needs to be done in a few minutes."

The deep desire to find fast and effective relief is understandable, but this is not what João's work stands for. He does not want to be cast in the role of a magician offering instant healing.

João de Deus recognizes that the symptoms of illness are part of a life problem that needs to be resolved. Spirits working through João can fertilize the seeds of health and well-being. The loving community of the Casa, which includes the entitys' work, may in fact be a kind of Miracle Grow—a substance which stimulates rapid, healthy growth. However, each person needs to be willing to take in the nurturing and change his or her life, and stop feeding the negativity which gave life to the illness in the first place.

Time is necessary. Time to rest, to reflect, to meditate, to be with others seeking healing, to care for one another. Time to listen to one's own sources of guidance—whether that be God, one's heart, a guardian spirit, or what you will. It is not unusual for people coming to Abadiania to stay for weeks. It is recommended that you stay a minimum of two weeks or more, to allow time for surgery and recovery. Work with yourself, the entities associated with João de Deus and your own sources of guidance continues wherever you are for months after your trip to Abadiania is over.

Taking the Work Home

You are encouraged to make the necessary changes in your life to support your healing when you return home. The important elements of continuing the work are: eating a wholesome diet, following dietary restrictions as necessary, having adequate rest, taking sufficient time to meditate and continue to align with what you consider Spirit. Dedication to this regime is especially important for those who need to return, as the herbs help build your body, and the meditation helps heal your mind in preparation for further surgery. It takes time for tissues to heal and cells to regenerate.

I believe that the greatest lessons to learn at the Casa involve how to take responsibility for your own recovery. The entities can only do their part, a large percentage of the healing work is up to each individual, whether you are returning or not. Many things influence the recovery rate including your karma, i.e., if you have been less than compassionate with others, and have harmed others to serve your own selfish ends, you may need to make amends to those whom you have hurt, or do volunteer work as a way of making amends to those no longer living. Having a positive attitude to life and relating to your fellow human beings is intrinsic to healing. Some may need to change their environment to support a more positive way of life.

You do not need to be a "religious" or "spiritual" person to go to Abadiania, or to make use of the healing available there. A will to get better, to take responsibility for your illness and make changes in your life is all that is required. João said "Those who travel great distances to come here already believe, even if they do not think they do."

Illustration:
Angel sculptures suspended from ceiling of the National Cathedral in Brasilia

PART SIX: WHERE DO WE GO FROM HERE?

artin Mosquera has been working very closely with João since 1998. He heads up the team of translators who facilitate the consultations between João-in-Entity and internationals who do not speak Portuguese. Martin speaks Spanish, Portuguese and English. I asked him to share his perspective on the Casa with me. We chose to sit on the second floor terrace of the Inn he manages, looking out over a large red bougainvillea, to the streets of Abadiania below us. From time to time Martin's seven year old son, Lucas, sprang up the spiral stairs for some attention. Martin's wife, Fernanda, remained downstairs attending to their baby and household tasks. Martin told me:

The entities who represent the Light, and their workers, are drawn to the Casa de Dom Inácio. They attend to requests; they help us connect more fully to God; and they want to share with health care professionals what they know about healing.

Abadiania is a unique and powerful energy spot on the earth. The entities want us to know that we are Spirit first. This will prepare us for eternal life, so we see physical death as a transition to further life and further growth. Then, we won't be so impatient while we are here on earth. We can wait for our food or our water. We will become more compassionate and more tolerant of others.

The Entity has said, 'There is a lot of transformation going on now. There is a big battle between the light and the dark forces.' The work at the Casa is purification. The entities come here to be close to us. They see things we don't see. They help us to open our hearts. *They help us to see that we are one being and there is one religion, which is called Love.* They help us to integrate that all is possible if we do it with God.

Some people who come here ask for a teaspoon full of the pure love, some ask for oceans. The entities give what we ask for. When visitors go home, they take their gifts with them to their communities. In this way we are assisting in the detoxification of the aura of the planet.

I felt inspired by what Martin said, and grateful that he had found words to describe the mysterious workings of the Casa. It is not an easy task to try to put the value of the Casa into words. People have varying degrees of acceptance for a place like the Casa, seemingly so different than our normal world.

After my return from my first trip to the Casa de Dom Inácio in April, 2001, members of our group

"They help us to see that we are one being and there is one religion, which is called Love."

shared our experience at an informal gathering at our local Universalist-Unitarian Church. When we told stories of healings we saw and healings we personally experienced, people were amazed, even incredulous.

There were a few who wanted to go to see the Entity's work with their own eyes. They intuitively felt it was real and were drawn to it. They nodded quietly during the presentation and later spoke to us privately.

The most vocal were agitated by our stories. One man, very ambivalent about taking in what he had heard, inquired insistently, almost belligerently: "What do you suggest I take with me from this meeting?" He was anxious to find some way to categorize João—a man doing successful surgery without antiseptics, anesthesia, or medical training. He wanted to either find a way that João in Entity would fit into the world he held as "real" — or to dismiss our stories.

Human beings find it very difficult to see or think about something they have previously called non-existent or impossible. William James, psychologist and philosopher, once said," If there is anything [that] human history demonstrates, it is the extreme slowness with which the academic and critical mind acknowledges facts to exist [that] present themselves as wild facts, with no stall or pigeonhole, or as facts [that] threaten to break up the accepted system."

This hesitation to accept what is foreign applies to the non-academic mind as well. It has been said that when the first English ship arrived on the coast of North America, the indigenous people could not see it, even though it was very visible and took up a lot of space in the harbor. The massive ship was simply outside their reality. It was an impossibility.

Present a 100 foot long sailing vessel to people who have only seen canoes and, one response will be dogged denial: "Large ships don't exist. Only canoes and rafts exist." People confronted with things outside their "reality" often deny what they are presented with or get irritated with the first person who steps on shore out of the dory, and points back to the ship lying in the harbor. "He must be lying or trying to trick me. Maybe he is crazy. White people, a new language, sharp metal instruments, sailing ships — it's all too new."

I don't know if this particular story about the American Indians is completely true...it may be largely apocryphal. However, there are many stories like it which illustrate the same point. The first man who announced that the world was round and not flat was considered out of his mind and publicly humiliated. Bringing a new vessel, or a new paradigm, into the harbor doesn't mean you will be seen or well received.

Doctors Wanting to Change

As awareness of the successes of spiritist centers in Brazil spreads, more of us will want to explore and/or implement aspects of Kardecist Spiritism into our own personal healing or health care practice.

Doctors do not need to align with benevolent spirits, put angels on duty in the wards, or take medium's training, in order to align with spiritist healing practices. Even if angels do exist, few of us currently have the eyes, ears and heart to communicate or align with them. It is better to take modest steps in our explorations. We need to first open to new possibilities and new viewpoints. Reading will help us reexamine ways in which we have previously kept the door closed on spiritual healing, as well as explore new potentials.

Larry Dossey, MD, was the co-chairperson of the Panel on Mind/Body Interventions of the Office of Alternative Medicine at the National Institute of Health from 1992-94. This office evolved into the NCCAM. He is currently the Executive Editor of "Alternative Therapies in Health and Medicine," a peer-review journal. His book, *Reinventing Medicine*, offers a conceptual framework for an "Era 3" or "Eternity" medicine which utilizes prayer and intuition alongside other forms of physical and body/mind interventions. Carolyn Myss, a reporter/publisher turned medical intuitive, offers audio-tape presentations, lectures and workshops in which people can learn to access their psychic abilities. Two psychiatrists, Judith Orloff (author of *Second Sight*) and Mona Lisa Schulz (author of *Awakening Intuition*,) help professionals to acknowledge, trust, and develop their intuitive skills to improve health care. Psychologist, Frank Lawlis, author of *Transpersonal Medicine*, interviews many of our most pioneering practitioners who are redefining health care to include the spiritual dimensions.

Narada, interviewed in Part Four, suggests that physicians return to the roots of their humanity, as well as the origins of their oath in becoming doctors:

Hippocrates told doctors, 'Heal Thyself.' I think he meant that doctors need to fully recognize that they are something other than the false ego. They are something more than their body, the color of their skin,

119

"If physicians and health professionals want to become more effective, they need to focus on getting in touch with their own spiritual consciousness."

their advanced education, their social status, their prestigious profession, their bank account, their success. They are, in fact, spiritual beings who need to fully connect with their spiritual intentions in order to help others become more whole, more at peace with themselves.

If physicians and health professionals want to become more effective, they need to focus on getting in touch with their own spiritual consciousness. They need to work towards manifesting Christ consciousness, that is, the intention to truly care for each person as if that person is our own brother...to truly be a dedicated servant of mankind and womankind. When physicians act with love and compassion in this way, resonating with their patients, feeling the deep connection, then they will help patients heal and cure.

Reading and personal work are two ways to move into a new paradigm of medicine. Another avenue is exploring modifications of therapeutic modalities which have been remodeled to include spiritual perspectives. For example, a pioneering psychiatrist, Brian Weiss, has been exploring past-life therapy through clinical hypnotherapy. One needs only be open to the *possibility* of reincarnation, to al-low spiritual perspectives to enter into more conventional therapy. Weiss finds that patients do not need to believe in Spiritism to have experiences involving past lives in which they let go of lifelong chronic pain and/or phobias. His success has given other practitioners encouragement to explore managing pain and phobias from a more spiritist perspective. More workshops and conferences are assisting health practitioners to integrate the new paradigm into their practices.

Dr. Richard Sandore, interviewed in Part Three, says, "When the healer is ready, the client will appear." When health practitioners open their own eyes to what is possible in healing, outside of their conventional training, they will be called on to use their vision. This happened with Dr. Erica Elliott, also interviewed in Part Three. Shortly after she returned from her transformative trip to the Casa de Dom Inácio, she was asked to do energetic healing work by her clients. This was very new for her. Six months later she designed a weekend workshop addressing the concept of illness as a call for spiritual growth.

If you are confronting an illness now

I expect that there will be many readers of this book who are ill and looking for perspective on their illness and treatment protocol. Many of you have cancer, feel ambivalent about conventional medical treatments, and are exploring complementary medical procedures.

In Parts Three and Four, both doctors and patients recommend going to the Casa de Dom Inácio for healing. They all say that their trips there were beneficial. I included these testimonies to illustrate the benefits of spiritist healing, but not to say that people *must* go to Abadiania to be healed of their illness. Just as important is to bring Abadiania and Brazilian spiritist centers into your own health management. The healing that takes place at spiritist centers makes use of many elements. Many of these elements are accessible to us in our home communities.

Donna Moseman, who tells about her confrontation with cancer in Part Four, clearly defined building blocks of her healing process. She recognized that she had to be very *honest with herself,* to get to the bare bones truth of why she wanted to live, before she could harness her strength to combat her cancer. By engaging her own personal truth, she could then manage her time and her energy to support her healing, without getting overly distracted by bending to the needs and expectations of others. Her soli-

tude in Abadiania provided her with the time for that personal confrontation, as well as a more *direct relationship with God*, which she sees as central to healing. Donna went on to allow herself to open to *the real possibility that benevolent spirits were working with her* in her home in Lebanon, New Hampshire, just as they were with her in Abadiania, Brazil. This was a new experience for her, opening her dramatically to the non-local potential of spiritual healing. Donna also chose an allopathic physician who was well-versed in western medicine as well as willing to support her own direction in complementary care. In a sense, Donna and her doctors created their own version of *"Integrative Medicine,"* because Donna felt free to coordinate with her physician about every mode of treatment. Thus, they were an aligned team, holding no secrets from each other, choosing together which health resources to employ. Finally, Donna continued *studying spiritual texts as well as doing her own spiritual practice*, activating the awareness that the life of the spirit in each of us is bigger than the passage of this life and its circumstances. This helped her identify with *the evolution of her spirit* during this life and beyond it into a future. Donna feels very strongly that her *community of friends and family* was the most important on-going aspect of her healing. She felt surrounded by love and support by people of all ages. She also worked with people in her area who were excellent at energy work and spiritual healing.

One thing that the Casa provides, which does not happen regularly in our neighborhoods, is active participation in an international, inter-generational group of individuals who are confronting serious illnesses or physical conditions. Healing is amplified when people who are ill get together in a supportive environment to share their struggles and their epiphanies, to pray together and pray for each other. Dean Ornish, MD, author, clinical professor at the University of California Medical School in San Francisco, and founder of Preventive Medicine Research Institute, is a member of the White House Commission on Complementary and Alternative Medicine Policy. He was the first to prove that heart disease is reversible by changing diet and lifestyle. The most important lifestyle changes he suggests are opening our hearts to one another and creating community. Drugs and surgery remove symptoms. They don't treat the underlying causes which often include a large component of loneliness, depression and isolation. When the causes are not handled, people return again to their disease states. This is personally difficult as well as an enormous financial burden for individuals, insurance companies, and medicare programs.[1]

Clinical studies continue to show that prayer has a very healing impact. The MANTRA project at Duke University is headed up by cardiologist Dr. Mitchell Krucoff and nurse practitioner, Susan Craven. Their results show that heart patients who receive prayer have 50 to 100 % fewer side effects than those patients treated with medicines, but not prayed for.

Thus, an essential ingredient for healing which we can create within our own communities is being with others who are also on a healing journey. Communicating with others takes us out of our loneliness and isolation. Connecting with physicians, disclosing our use of complementary and alternative therapies, can potentially enhance our relationship as well as facilitate a more integrated treatment protocol. (Most complementary and integrative therapies are neither disclosed nor discussed with medical doctors.)[2] Connecting with others who are ill presents opportunities to laugh, to get outside of the negative thoughts and fears that often accompany disease, to affirm the spiritual connections which we have because we are human beings. Mauro, the man interviewed in Part Four who had suffered from AIDS, continued to visit the Casa de Dom Inácio every forty-five days after his health returned. He shifted his role in the community from being a person who needed support to a person who was providing support to others. His service gave him continual contact with the Casa and his friends there who had seen him through his illness. Prayer and meditation continued consistently. The ever-changing community of people on healing journeys helped him expand his commitment to a lifestyle of good health and charity.

Becoming a Healer or Starting a Center

Many of those who had been healed at the Casa decided to continue their involvement there, as did Mauro, and/or to cultivate their abilities as healers. Martin (quoted at the beginning of this Part) asked João what meditation would be helpful for someone who wants to strengthen their abilities as a medium. The medium, João, suggested:

> Go first to the beginning of Creation and the Creator of that creation. It is infinite love, infinite intelligence and wisdom. Bring that energy into you. It will also provide you with protection.
>
> Then, go inside the planet, into the fire that is inside the planet. Bring that fire into you. It will burn away all that is impure in you. The earth is also like a mother. It knows everything about you. You can not lie to this energy.
>
> Next, with your spiritual teacher and his or her lineage, go directly to God and ask for what you want for your friends, family, or clients. You may ask for blessings, for healing, for clarity, etc.
>
> Do not ask for a specific Entity to be channeled through you. God will send the right Entity to you.

Over and over, the Entity has said to people—

> It depends only on you. How far you go in becoming a medium or working in spiritual realms depends on you. We have to work very hard on our-

selves spiritually to acquire what is necessary to work in spirit. It is demanding. It asks of you that you continue your work of purification; that you let go of egoistic desires and become a vessel through which spirit can work. It is God that is doing the work. He will use you as the instrument you are. You must also ask for what you want. God will come to you *only* when you make the request.

João, the man, was asked in November, 2000, if anyone can perform the kind of healings which he does. João answered, "My gift is a gift from God. With Him all things are possible. If you pray to be able to do the kind of healing I do, you can receive it." Next João was asked if there will be anything like the Casa in other countries. He responded, "If God wants it—then it will go to many places." To me, it follows: if it is God's will, many others will become able to do spiritist healing.

Taking our first steps to practice Spiritist healing is not done by immediately trying to mimic João, or perform the work of a medium *without sustained effort in building skills and without the profound dedication to this mission which João de Deus personifies*. It is irresponsible to go home and perform surgery without anesthesia, just because some inner voice told you to, or because you know that someone else can do it successfully. More appropriate action would be to contact a reputable school of healing, such as the Barbara Brennan School of Healing.[3] This school offers four year training programs and makes referrals to their graduates who live in many areas of the world.

> Each spirit is destined to possess all possible aptitudes; but, in order to progress, he must possess one sole and unitary will.
> —from Kardec's "The Spirits' Book"

It is not a good idea to expect that everyone who calls themselves a spiritual healer has the same capacity or skill level. We don't expect all doctors to equally competent just because they have all earned an MD or a doctorate. We know some will be better at certain specialties than others. The same is true of spiritual healers. We can't expect that all spiritual healers will exhibit the same range of skills, or have the same gifts. Some will be better at their specialty than others. Healers have unique gifts. The Brazilian Spiritist Federation in San Paulo lists 128 different kinds of specialties practiced by mediums.

I had a powerful experience at the Casa which helped open the door to understanding the resources of a healer. On September 19, 2001, I was in the Entity's current room meditating when it was announced that Dom Inácio, (the patron saint of the Casa, and the individual for whom it was named), would be incorporating in João the next day. Incorporation of Dom Inácio's energy is particularly demanding on João and he needs many people to meditate in service to the work on days when this happens. The next day Anneke Visser (interviewed in Part Three) and I meditated together in the Entity's room with the intention of helping the Entity. For more than three hours we each had the experience that as soon as we had energy to offer, it was used for healing others. Both of us felt empty, totally empty... and, simultaneously full because, in our willingness to be of service, all that was left was our bodies being used as vessels through which streamed the healing force of Love. I now understand more deeply the phrase, "By giving, we receive."

Having profound experiences of healing at the Casa inspires many people to consider starting centers like the Casa. Setting up a center in your country does not mean it has to have all the elements of the Casa de Dom Inácio or any other spiritist center in Brazil. There is no prescription for how to start a center, like the Casa de Dom Inácio, except to fol-low the promptings which come from your own intuition. Anica Visser , for one, feels called to set up a center in Europe, most likely in Spain. She wants people to feel comfortable outdoors all year round. Anneke will have many practitioners representing various forms of complementary medicine, as well as optional study of the Course in Miracles.

Brazil: A Leader in the 21st century

The promise of a new kind of health care is emerging from people all over the world, but a powerful symbol for this is a structure in Brasilia, Brazil's capital. Templo da Boa Vontade, The Temple of Good Will (TGW,) was built in Brasilia, in 1989. Close to seventy feet high, this temple was envisioned by Paiva Netto, as a place of meditation and retreat. The temple walls enclose a large open space. On the center of the ground floor is a spiral walkway. There are no rituals associated with the temple. At all hours of the day, individuals of all faiths come to sit quietly and/or walk the spiral, as a walking meditation, if they choose. The spiral begins with a dark marble path, symbolizing the work of purification that needs to be done leading to the center and a white marble path leading out from the center, symbolizing the path of light which can be walked after the work is done. Above the altar, a handsome table, is an artistic rendition of the four elements: earth, air, fire and water. Outside the temple is an eternal flame representing the solidarity of all people of good will. Underneath the temple floor, lit by sidewall skylights, is the Egyptian Room, a room for silent meditation, beautifully decorated with Egyptian art.

TGW sits in a grassy area in the middle of the city, across the street from a cluster of Brasilia's finest hospitals, and thus available to patients and health-care workers. TGW is sometimes called the Temple of Unrestricted Ecumenism because it was erected for the well-being of terrestrial humans as well as spiritual beings, both of whom are in the process of evolution. The visionary behind the philosophy of this center, Alziro Zarur, believed that when humans understand that their origins are spiritual, that there is no death but eternal life, that God is within them, then they can construct a better and happier world. *According to Netto and Zarur, we are all brothers and sisters under the same father, God, a synonym for Love.*

Forums of humanitarian and spiritual interest are hosted by TGW in the World Parliament of Ecumenical Fraternity, also named the Third Millennium Forum, adjacent to the temple. Inaugurated

in 1994, this five story building has become a central meeting place for dialogues about *spiritually-based medicine* amongst other topics. The plenary room seats five hundred, with a panoramic view of Brasilia, eight booths for simultaneous translation, and a room for the press. Two other auditoriums hold seats for two hundred and one hundred, respectively. The Student's Quarters provides computers for internet access for more than twelve thousand students per month. A reception area is available for cultural events. A restaurant and snack bar serve visitors and students on a daily basis. This building is a meeting space for all of us who are participating in bringing a new vi-

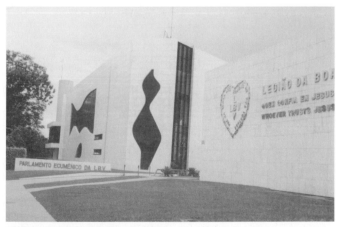

World Parliament of Ecumenical Fraternity in Brasilia

sion down to earth which is based on interconnectedness and love.

The first structure to be erected in Brasilia, a city built in the late 1950s on nothing but architectural design and raw land, was a small marble pyramid commemorating the vision of an Italian priest and educator. This man, Dom Bosco, prophesied in 1883 that a new civilization would arise on the site of present day Brasilia. Brasilia was thus dubbed "The Capital of the Third Millennium," a worldy title for the new location of a Capital in what is still referred to as a "third world country." A larger building in the center of the capital now commemorates the value of Dom Bosco's vision. The Sanctuary of Dom Bosco, whose walls are made almost entirely of blue and violet stained-glass, is one of Brasilia's most beautiful churches.

Anneke Visser and I spent three hours at the Temple of Good Will, just a few weeks after the terrorist annihilation of the World Trade Center in New York City. Standing in the center, between the path of darkness and the path of light, I prayed for our world. The visions of Dom Bosco and Paivo Netto, transformed into the building in which I stood, were a comfort and an inspiration. Yes, there are people,

and there have been people in past centuries, who see what must be done to encourage a human culture built on interconnectedness, balance and equality.

We are not in balance when 4.5% of the world's population, that is North America, uses 30% of the world's resources.[4] How easy it is to lose our balance as we compete for, or protect, our material well-being. How easy it has become to forget our spiritual roots, our spiritual alliances and our spiritual destiny. Most recently, we look for the terrorists who attack the symbols of our way of life; we forget to listen compassionately to the problems of other countries who are in the backwash of our over-consumption. We fight for the right to continue our materialistic life, rather than come to the negotiating table to discuss how to share resources and be stewards of the earth. We fear letting go of our old habits even when those habits are taking us to poor health, depression, impoverished health care systems, environmental degradation, economic decline and war.

Perhaps this is the terror we need to vanquish: our fear of change...our fear of meeting all human beings as brothers and sisters...our fear of direct connection to spiritual realms...our fear of dissolving what has kept us separate from spiritual alliances.

When *these* fears no longer run wild—when they are contained—then we will be in a position to create a world without terrorism. Then, we can create genuine international alliances which honor the unique spirit of each culture...world judiciary systems which uphold basic human rights...a world economy which values sustaining the earth's resources... and a health care system which fully recognizes that health is a community and spiritually based issue.

For me, The Temple of Good Will is a symbol of our transition to this new way of living, inspiring my participation, and helping me feel connected to others who share my intention. Perhaps the temple can be this symbol for you as well. Paivo Netto said, "More important than erecting a material temple is to raise the Temple of the Living God in human hearts. It was necessary to come forth with a human-spiritual reconciling symbol that is to guide men on their path toward Fraternity in the Third Millennium."

Temple of Good Will

As new as this temple is, the seed for its creation was there in Kardec's "The Spirits' Book," written in 1861. To his question: "Will progress ultimately unite all the peoples of the earth into a single nation?" The reply:

No, not into a single nation; that is impossible, because the diversities of climate give rise to diversities of habits and of needs that constitute diverse nationalities, each of which will always need laws appropriate to its special habits and needs. But charity knows nothing of latitudes, and makes no distinction between the various shades of human color; and when the law of God shall be everywhere the basis of human law, the law of charity will be practiced between nation and nation as between man and man, and all will then live in peace and happiness, because no one will attempt to wrong his neighbor, or to live at his expense.

128

Glossary

Acupuncture— a medical practice that treats illness or provides local anesthesia by the insertion of needles at specified sites of the body.

Allopathic—pertaining to a method of treating disease by the use of agents (e.g. drugs and surgical interventions) that produce effects different from those of the disease treated.

Angel—a messenger or minister of God. A highly evolved, pure spirit who serves the evolution and protection of sentient beings and maintains universal harmony. According to Kardec, angels "exercise a sovereign command over all spirits inferior to themselves, aid them in accomplishing the work of their purification, and assign to each of them a mission proportioned to the progress already made by them."

Automatic writing—(aka psychography in Brazil) a process whereby a medium allows his/her hand to be moved by a disembodied spirit for the purpose of communicating with human beings through written messages.

Channel—(n.) known in Brazil as "one who has incorporated an entity;" a medium who allows a disembodied spirit to use his/her body for the purpose of serving others through inspired speech or healing action.

Channeling—(v.) allowing a disembodied spirit to use one's body to communicate specific information to other human beings.

Clairaudience—(n.; clairaudient, adj.) a psychic gift which enables a medium to hear subtle perceptions beyond the limitations of the normal, physical five senses.

Clairsentience—(n.; clairsentient, adj.) a psychic gift which enables a medium to accurately feel what others are feeling in sensation and emotion without prior information or evidence.

Clairvoyance—(n.; clairvoyant, adj.) a psychic gift which allows a medium to see subtle perceptions beyond the limitations of the normal physical sense of vision. This might include seeing energy fields, seeing visions of the future, seeing what someone has experienced in the past, or seeing with x-ray vision into the body.

Complementary Health Care—protocols formerly outside the scope of allopathic health care. Complementary health care includes, but is not limited to, nutrition, chiropractic, acupuncture, massage, herbal remedies, Yoga therapy.

Curandeiro—a word used in South America to refer to a medicine person aligned with indigenous traditions having a strong relationship to the earth. Curandeiros are reputed to have powers to disidentify with material reality and direct subtle and powerful energies towards others with either harmful or beneficial results.

Current (ref. "sitting in current")—the energy created by many mediums sitting silently together with the intention to amplify healing through being open to highly evolved spiritual energies.

Demon—an entity who serves the most base human instincts, generating lust, greed, fear, anger, and/or destruction. A demon's intention to help others evolve spiritually is almost completely buried under negative intentions. Kardec writes: "If demons exist, it is in your low world, and in other worlds of similar degree, that they are to be found. They are the human hypocrites who represent a just God as being cruel and vindictive, and who imagine that they make themselves agreeable to Him by the abominations they commit in His name."

Deposession—a practice of exorcising negative spirits from a physical place or a physical person.

Disobsession—a practice of exorcising negative spirits from a person who feels victim to obsessions and compulsions.

Doctrine of Spiritism—information systematically collated by Allen Kardec from channels who received information from highly evolved disembodied spirits. This doctrine answers many fundamental questions such as "Why are humans on earth,? "What should we do with our lives," "Are disembodied spirits available to help us in our evolution,?" "How can we define God and Christ's relationship to God,?" and "Is death something to be feared?"

Energy Body—energy which both sustains and protects a human body. Some part of this is universal and some part is highly personal, interwoven with attitudes, values and viewpoints of the individual.

Energy Work—a practice whereby a health practitioner attends to the well-being of the body through balancing energies.

Entity (also Disembodied Entity)-a spirit which has formerly had a body but now exists in a spiritual realm invisible to most human beings. This spirit is continuing to work on its spiritual evolution which might include preparing for another lifetime in a body.

> **Negative Entity**—a disembodied entity motivated by bad intentions

> **Positive Entity**—a disembodied entity motivated by intentions to assist others in their spiritual evolution

Exorcism—an event whereby an individual is assisted to release his/her attachment to negative entities and/or negative thought forms (obsessions and compulsions.)

Extrasensory perception (ESP)—perceptions which reach farther than the limitations of the five physical senses—hearing, seeing, touching, tasting and smelling. Often called "the sixth sense," ESP is the subject of the study of parapsychology. It is also the vehicle used by mediums to diagnose and treat patients without having to rely on objective physical assessments of symptoms and statistical data.

Hari Krishna movement—a religious movement originating in India designed to assist people in their spiritual evolution through prayer, service, chanting, study, and devotional life.

Healing at a Distance—healing that takes place through the agency of one or more healers who are not in the physical presence of the patient.

Holy Spirit—the ineffable, most powerful energy of creation, having the qualities of truth, creativity, infinite knowledge, grace, pure awareness and compassion. This universal energy is perceived as an aspect of God for Christians. Particular elements of this energy are named diversely in various cultures, e.g. Buddha, Dharma, Shakti, Shiva, Allah.

Homeopathy—a method of treating disease by minute doses of drugs/organic substances that in a healthy person would produce symptoms similar to those of the disease.

Immuno-therapy—medical treatment designed to enhance the immune system.

Incorporate (v.)— to deliberately invite an entity to use one's body for a specific purpose, e.g. John of God incorporates Dom Inácio for healing others.

Invisible surgery— healing effected by an outside agent that is done inside the body of the patient without the use of physical instruments or opening the body through surgery. Prayer is often used in invisible surgery to summon positive entities and angels who promote healing of the body and mind without invasive procedures.

Kardec, Allan—the author of the doctrine of Spiritism.

Kardecist—of or pertaining to the writing or doctrine of Allan Kardec.

Karma—the law of cause and effect as it applies to spiritual evolution, i.e. an action motivated by bad intention causes a reaction which feeds negativity. An action motivated by loving intention causes an effect which feeds spiritual evolution for everyone involved.

Kelly Clamp—metal scissor-like device with a forty degree angle toward the top used in medical procedures.

Laying on of Hands—the practice of directing healing energy through one's hands for the purpose of facilitating health and well-being in the recipient. E.g. Reiki practitioners intentionally ask that the energy of the Holy Spirit come through their hands to empower healing. Their hands may or may not touch the body of the recipient.

Medium—a sensitive, a person with some psychic ability/abilities, a person serving as an instrument for some supernatural agency. A person who has the power to perceive and/or communicate with those in spiritual realms.

Medium's training—training through study and practice to elicit and hone skills of being a medium. This training is offered in many spiritist centers and is supervised by mediums who are have demonstrated their expertise.

Miracle—(from Webster's Dictionary) an extraordinary occurrence that surpasses all known human powers or natural forces and is ascribed to a divine or supernatural cause, esp. to God.

Osteopathy-a system of medical practice emphasizing the manipulation of muscles and bones to promote structural integrity and the relief of certain disorders.

Parapsychology—the study of psi phenomena (see below).

Passes (energetic)—particular ways in which a healer sends energy to a patient through hand movements above and/or around the body. Passes infrequently touch the physical body.

Perfection—the goal of spiritual evolution refers to a state of consciousness recognizable through bliss, compassion, happiness, wisdom and a desire to serve others. Spiritists believe that working toward perfection through purification and selfless service is the most important activity of life.

Peri-spirit—the semi-material envelope linking the spirit and the body during life. It survives the transition we call death. This envelope carries the imprint of previous life lessons learned as well as aspirations for the future. It is the means by which the spirit acts upon matter and that matter acts upon the spirit. The peri-spirit can assume any form that the spirit may choose to give it.

Phrenology— the study of the conformation of the skull based on the belief that it is indicative of mental faculties and character.

Protocol—a plan for carrying out a patient's treatment regimen.

Psi Phenomena/psychic phenomena—events related to acquiring knowledge without cues from the external senses, often related to "the sixth sense." Examples: mental telepathy, automatic writing, healing at a distance, channeling, psychokinesis, clairsentience, clairvoyance and clairaudience.

Psychokinesis—a direct energetic influence exerted on a physical system which creates movement or inner change without the use of any physical instruments; e.g. mind over matter.

Radiotherapy—treatment of disease by radioactive substances

Soul—an incarnate spirit, that part of human intelligence which survives death and continues to live in a realm invisible to most humans.

Spirit—a soul before it unites with the body, that part of the human which survives death and continues to live in a realm invisible to most humans. Spirits assume a fleshly body in order to effect their purification and enlightenment. On the lower end of evolution are spirits who are destructive, obsessive, ignorant, never satisfied and lost in repetitive negative thinking and behavior. On the higher levels are spirits who are wise, happy and compassionate.

Spiritism—a spiritual movement which makes use of benevolent intradimensional dialogue between humans, God and spirits to facilitate well-being.

Spirit Realm—a distinct realm of life, unrelated to physical time and space, peopled by those who are between lives, still able to influence those in body, and preparing themselves for their next step in evolution. There are diverse levels of evolution in the disembodied spirits who populate this realm.

Spiritual Anesthesia—a relief of painful sensation made possible by spirits. This form of anesthesia is often experienced by people undergoing surgery at the Casa de Dom Inácio. Spiritual anesthesia makes it possible to stand, think rationally, and communicate clearly while undergoing surgery.

Spiritualism—a philosophy emphasizing the spiritual aspect of being, allowing for the possibility that our spirits survive death.

Triage—the determination of priorities for action in medical issues

Unconscious medium—a medium who enters an altered state of consciousness, as if his personality is asleep, while he or she channels a disembodied entity for the purpose of assisting others. For example, John of God may have been channeling for 12 hours, performing surgeries, consulting with hundreds of people, and saying prayers—none of which he remembers in his normal state of consciousness.

NOTES

PART ONE

1. Pellegrino-Estrich, R. (2001)" The Miracle Man: The Life Story of João de Deus." Cairns, Australia: Triad Publishers
2. Ibid.
3. Savaris, AA (1997) Curas Paranormais Realizadas Por João Teixeira de Farias. Curitiba, Brazil: Curitiba Press
4. Fouts, D. (2001) "Your Battle Against Aging and Disease," audio-taped lecture. Available through Dupli-Pack Phone: 888-443-1979. Dr. Fouts is a Chiropractor specializing in Radiology, Orthopedics, and Nutrition. Since 1995, Dr. Fouts has extensively researched the medical literature on Glyconutrients to help people with chronic degenerative and auto immune diseases significantly improve their health conditions.
5. Eisenberg DM, Davis RB, Ettner SL, Appel S, Wilkey S, Van Rompay, M, Kessler R, "Trends in Alternative Medicine Use in the United States, 1990-1997," in *Journal of the American Medical Association*, 280 (1998): 1569-75.
6. National Center for Complementary and Alternative Medicine, (September, 2000) "Expanding Horizons in Healthcare: Five Year Strategic Plan, 2001-2005." Bethesda, MD: NCCAM
7. Eisenberg et al., Ibid.
8. Astin, John (1998) "Why Patients Use Alternative Medicine: Results of a National Survey" in the *Journal of the American Medical Association*, 279 (1998):1548-53.

PART TWO

1. "No Reino Dos Espiritos (In The Realm of Spirits)" in *Veja*, January 4th, 1984, pg. 40.
2. Hess, David J. (1994). Samba in the Night: Spiritism in Brazil. NYC: Columbia University Press

PART THREE

1. Edgar Cayce's Association for Research and Enlightenment was founded in 1931 to research transpersonal subjects such as holistic health and contemporary spirituality. See www.are-cayce.com
2. Dossey, L. (1993) Healing Words, San Francisco: HarperSanFrancisco, pp 243-247
3. Ibid., Healing Words

Part Four

1. Dossey, L. (1993) Healing Words, San Francisco: HarperSanFrancisco, pp 211-235

Part Six

1. Ornish, Dean (2000) "Health" in Imagine: What America Could be in the 21st Century. NYC: New American Library
2. Eisenberg DM, Davis RB, Ettner SL, Appel S, Wilkey S, Van Rompay, M, Kessler R, "Trends in alternative medicine use in the United States, 1990-1997: results of a follow-up national survey. *Journal of the American Medical Association*, 1998; 280:1569-75
3. Barbara Brennan School of Healing, has a website (www.barbarabrennan.com) which describes its programs, and lists referrals to healers around the world, as well as upcoming events, speaking engagements and workshops. See "Resources" at the back of this book.
4. Hawken, Paul (2000), "Possibilities" in Imagine: What America Could be in the 21st Century. NYC: New American Library

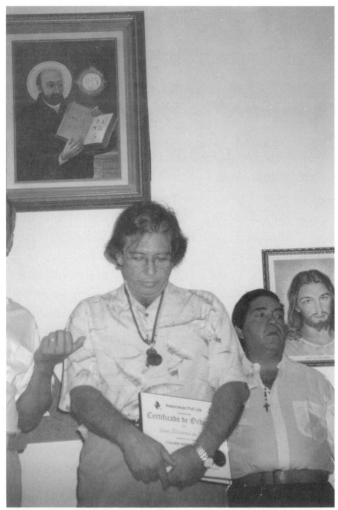

João Teixara de Faria after being ordained as a healer in the Full Life Church by Ron Roth

RESOURCES

In and Around Abadiania:

The Casa Grounds, Shops, and Treatment Facilities

Several outbuildings attached to the main assembly room serve visitors in various ways. A pharmacy sells containers of herb capsules, fulfilling prescriptions by the Entity. (Five bottles, the normal prescription, cost $20.) A concession for buying snacks and fresh juices is open every day the Entity is at the Casa. Another shop which sells water that has been blessed as well as souvenirs like crystals, T-shirts, rosaries, videos and books are open Wednesdays, Thursdays and Fridays. There is always one Casa staff-person capturing the daily work of the Casa on video. Copies of these videos are available for sale at minimal cost to anyone who requests them.

Bathroom facilities for men and women are kept up to the cleanliness standards of common public restrooms in the USA. A garden area, lawns and benches under flowering trees offer special spots for sitting, conversing or meditating.

For a fee of $10, one can have a "crystal bed" healing session in a private room lying on a bed over which seven crystals are held in a frame, aimed at the seven energy centers of the body. An attendant makes sure that the room is clean, the scheduling orderly, and the lights aimed to match the energy centers of each patient. For twenty minutes,

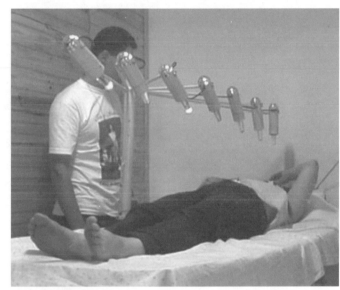

Crystal Bed Healing Session

gentle music is played and flashing lights filtered by various colors beam through the crystals onto the person lying on the bed. The effect is balancing and energizing.

The Entity prescribes the crystal room to some people as part of their treatment. One woman with very advanced breast cancer was on slow morphine drip continuously, but was still in a great deal of discomfort. The Entity prescribed crystal bed treatments only, usually six times per day, throughout her stay. She reported that the crystal treatments eliminated her pain completely.

Staying in the Community close to the Casa de Dom Inácio

There are several inns throughout the neighborhood around the Casa which offer rooms with private baths and three meals a day. These small hotels are clean. The food is wholesome. By North American standards, the prices are very modest. The inns charge about $15 per day for room and board. Taxis are available to assist people who can not walk the short distance to the Casa and back. Arrangements can also be made through the hotels for transfers to and from the airports.

Many of the inns are run by volunteers at the Casa who assist in the healing and recovery rooms as well as manage the business of their inns. They consider that their small hotels are like the wards of a large hospital—where beneficent entities come to work on their patients at all times of day and night.

All of the inns have phones and most have faxes. A few have computers. The only difficulty in making reservations and the arrangements with these small hotels is that few are run by English speaking people, and few travelers from abroad speak Portuguese.

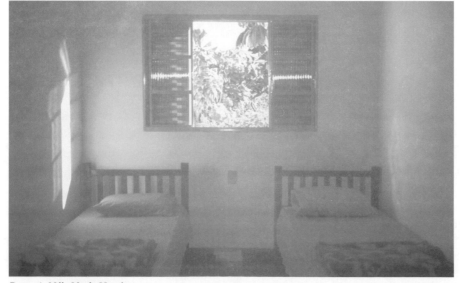
Room 1, Villa Verde Hotel

Food and Water

The food at all the inns is quite similar. In keeping with the dietary restrictions of the Casa for people who are taking herbs or convalescing after surgery: no pork, alcohol, fertilized eggs, non-organic bananas or pepper (black pepper, chili peppers of any kind, etc.) are served.

Lunch and dinner is usually the same. White rice and some form of beans are always served as well as salads or fresh vegetables. Although the food is repetitious it is easy to survive as a vegetarian. For meat-eaters, there is fish or chicken. Beef is available less frequently.

Breakfast is predictably the same each morning. Strong Brazilian coffee, with or without sugar. Yeasted white flour rolls. Butter. Tropical fruit jam. Farmer's cheese. Fresh fruit: pineapple, watermelon and papaya. Some inns also serve lunch meat at breakfast-time. Cake is considered a special breakfast food and is offered on weekend meals. Eggs may be available on request.

Bottled water, with or without carbonation, is kept chilled and available for an extra charge at each inn. Many visitors elect to purchase all their water at the Casa, because it has been blessed by the entities and is believed to be a significant part of the healing. People speak of minor problems being treated by just drinking the water. The Casa's bottled water is more expensive than water at the inns.

Massage

There are several massage practitioners available to visitors to Abadiania. Their work ranges from deep tissue massage which is highly physical and energizing to a more comforting, soothing body work. If you want to combine massage with the treatment you are doing with the Entity, it is strongly suggested you first ask permission of the Entity.

Logistics of Travel

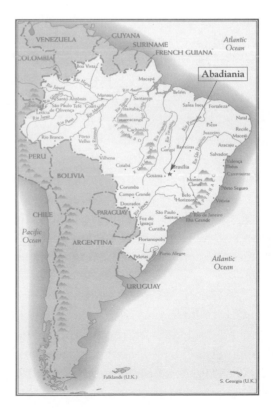

For practical information about traveling to the Casa de Dom Inácio, reserving accommodations at pousadas (inns), and arranging for taxi pickup at the airport:

www.friendsofthecasa.org

If web site addresses are not accessible: Send $2. and a self-addressed stamped envelope for a booklet of information to the following address:

JD Rabbit, 1577 Chase Brook Rd, Berlin, VT 05602 or contact JD by email: jdr@together.net

Brazilian American Cultural Club (BACC):

800-222-2746 has **blocks of seats on flights to Brazil** which they sell to individuals at more reasonable prices than most international travel agencies. They book dependable airlines and can also help with visas. You need to fly to Brasilia or Goiania airport. **You must have a visa.**

For a list of Certified Guides of the Casa with their contact information—go to: www.friendsofthe casa.org and click on the section for guides in the index. These people have offered their services. Each has different qualifications. It is highly useful to choose a guide who speaks flu-

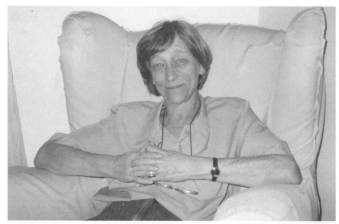

Julika Kiskos, PhD.

ent Portuguese, as well as one who has spent at least three months at the Casa and is, thus, familiar with the culture there. This will assist you in understanding your consultations with João—and assist João, and other Casa volunteers, in communicating effectively with you. Robert Pellegrino-Estrich and his wife, Catarina, have been taking large groups to visit the Casa de Dom Inácio since 1986. Catarina speaks Portuguese and is a healer in her own right.

Emma Bragdon leads trips to the Casa and to other spiritist centers in Brazil. These trips may include workshops with Julika Kiskos (fluent in Portuguese and English)—a Brazilian psychologist who has been involved with spiritist healing practices since 1975. For further information contact Emma Bragdon.

802-457-4915 or Email: EBragdon@aol.com
www.emmabragdon.com